# THE CTG IN PRACTICE

**Adam H Balen**
MB BS MRCOG

**John H Smith**
MA MB B.Chir MD MRCOG

**CHURCHILL LIVINGSTONE**
EDINBURGH LONDON MADRID MELBOURNE NEW YORK AND TOKYO 1992

CHURCHILL LIVINGSTONE
Medical Division of Longman Group UK Limited

Distributed in the United States of America by
Churchill Livingstone Inc., 650 Avenue of the Americas, New York,
N.Y. 10011, and by associated companies, branches and
representatives throughout the world.

© Longman Group UK Limited 1992

First published 1992

ISBN 0-443-04675-1

**British Library Cataloguing in Publication Data**
A catalogue record for this book is available from
the British Library.

Produced by Longman Singapore Publishers (Pte) Ltd
Printed in Singapore

*To Frances and Joanna*

We would like to thank Mrs Josephine Gorman, Senior Midwife Coordinator at the Central Middlesex Hospital, who encouraged the collection of cases as a labour ward training manual for the midwives and junior doctors.

# Foreword

It is a curious fact that the use of continuous electronic fetal heart rate monitoring (EFHRM) in maternity units remains as popular as ever despite many reports in the literature that its use has not resulted in any observed fall in perinatal mortality. The reasons for this paradox are complex and this is not the place to discuss them. However, it is certain that clinicians feel secure in the knowledge that an entirely normal trace is a very reliable sign that the fetus is in good condition despite adverse clinical features that suggest the contrary. Whatever the explanation, the reality is that nearly every maternity unit in Britain uses EFHRM, and it is essential that doctors and midwives working in these units know how to interpret the traces.

Adam Balen and John Smith have combined to produce an eminently practical, readable manual of cardiotocography in labour. The mixture of case presentations and FHR traces adds interest by highlighting the strengths and limitations of monitoring in labour. This strongly practical approach is supported by considerations of many other aspects of labour ward management, such as the use of partograms, the management of premature rupture of membranes and even a brief excursion into the problems for women who have had a ritual circumcision!

The authors rightly point to the limitations of EFHRM as a reliable predictor of fetal asphyxia when used as the final diagnostic index. They draw attention to the known increase in caesarean section rate that accompanies this practice. They recommend fetal blood sampling as a valuable adjunct to EFHRM as it increases diagnostic specificity and sensitivity. They also suggest that the time has come to reassess the policy of monitoring all women in labour. Perhaps the selection of the high risk baby is now so much improved that we can abandon universal monitoring and concentrate on women designated as high risk, but not everyone would agree with this view. However, for those who read this book, the acknowledgement that many issues surrounding the safety of the fetus are unresolved should encourage them to read further.

Finally the recent upsurge of medico-legal problems in obstetrics, most of which are related to labour ward practice, underlines the importance of all obstetricians and midwives having an agreed working knowledge and understanding of monitoring procedures. The finding by Ennis & Vincent (1990) that in one-third of perinatal deaths that came to the courts, the SHO lacked knowledge of how to interpret a CTG trace, makes this book compulsory reading for all who care for women in labour.

I congratulate the authors on their achievement and am sure that they will soon be preparing the next edition.

R W Beard
Professor, Department of Obstetrics & Gynaecology
St Mary's Hospital Medical School, London

Ennis M, Vincent C A 1990 Obstetric accidents: a review of 64 cases. British Medical Journal 300: 1365–1367

# Preface

In recent years there have been several advances in the technology for monitoring the fetus, both ante- and intrapartum. In the past, intermittent auscultation was performed using simple listening devices such as the Pinard stethoscope. Electronic devices (cardiotocographs) for recording the fetal heart rate are now widely used, whilst research continues in the development of techniques for assessing the other parameters of fetal physiology. When continuous intrapartum monitoring is necessary, the best method at present is a combination of cardiotocography and fetal blood sampling.

The cases in this book were collected over a year at the Central Middlesex Hospital, London. Unfortunately, fetal blood sampling was not available and so the cardiotocograph (CTG) alone was relied upon. Although it is now recognized that a measurement of fetal hypoxaemia and acidosis is an essential adjunct for the reliable interpretation of a CTG, 55% of units in the United Kingdom still lack these facilities. We therefore present a wide range of clinical situations which illustrate how safely to interpret the CTG when it is the only means of monitoring a fetus before and during labour. Also, we hope to demonstrate both how this technology can help the midwife and obstetrician—and how it can fail them. The last three cases are from St. Mary's Hospital, London. Here fetal blood sampling is available and these examples demonstrate that, whilst being a useful adjunct to the CTG, a fetal blood sample still does not provide all the answers.

Most books on fetal monitoring demonstrate brief examples of particular abnormalities which are difficult to relate to a clinical situation. In this book we present the histories of 25 pregnant women, together with a selection of CTG traces taken either antenatally or at various times during labour. We have also included the partogram in half of the cases, so that the CTGs can be seen in the context of the progress of labour. In addition to specific comments on aspects of fetal monitoring, we also discuss other aspects of labour ward care, together with practical advice that is not always to be found in conventional textbooks.

The book was initially designed for 'round table' teaching and discussion on the labour ward between a senior obstetrician or midwife and junior doctors and midwives in training. It is hoped that it is seen as a practical guide for all those involved in labour ward care.

Adam Balen and John Smith
London, 1992

# Abbreviations

| | | | | |
|---|---|---|---|---|
| ARM | artificial rupture of membranes | | LOP | left occipito-posterior |
| BP | blood pressure | | LOT | left occipito-transverse |
| BPP | biophysical profile | | Mec | meconium |
| BS | blood stained liquor | | NVD | normal vaginal delivery |
| CL | clear liquor | | OA | occipito-anterior |
| CPD | cephalopelvic disproportion | | OP | occipito-posterior |
| CTG | cardiotocogram | | P | para |
| Cx | cervix | | $pCO_2$ | partial pressure of carbon dioxide |
| ECG | electrocardiogram | | $pO_2$ | partial pressure of oxygen |
| EDD | estimated date of delivery | | ROA | right occipito-anterior |
| FBS | fetal blood sampling | | ROM | rupture of membranes |
| FSE | fetal scalp electrode | | ROP | right occipito-posterior |
| G | gravida | | ROT | right occipito-transverse |
| HIE | hypoxic–ischaemic encephalopathy | | SROM | spontaneous rupture of membranes |
| IUPC | intrauterine pressure catheter | | TOP | termination of pregnancy |
| IUD | intrauterine death | | UAI | uterine activity integral |
| LMP | last menstrual period | | USS | ultrasound scan |
| LOA | left occipito-anterior | | VE | vaginal examination |
| LOC | loss of contact | | | |

# Contents

# Introduction

The cardiotocograph (CTG) provides an indication of fetal well-being. *Cardio-* refers to heart rate and *toco-* to uterine contraction. Both are represented at the same time, the heart rate at the top of the trace and contractions at the bottom. The machinery used to measure these parameters employs either external transducers or internal electrodes. Whilst the fetal heart rate may be detected by either an external microphone or electrocardiogram (ECG), both are subject to interference; the microphone from the noise of maternal movement and the ECG from the maternal heart's intrinsic electrical activity. The most reliable method of recording the fetal heart activity is by an external ultrasound transducer which detects the reflected, or Doppler, shift of transmitted ultrasound waves. The external transducer is held in place by an elasticated belt around the maternal abdomen, and the contraction monitor is similarly placed. The heart monitor may be connected directly to the CTG machine, or, if telemetry is available, the signal may be transmitted to a central monitor, so allowing maternal mobility and hence greater comfort during the first stage of labour. An internal electrode may be used once the membranes have ruptured and the mother is in established labour; it is attached directly to the presenting fetal part—usually the head (see Case 19).

Fetal heart rate varies as a result of many factors, but heart rate is just one parameter of fetal physiology that alters during stress. The heart rate is monitored because it is easily detected and recorded, but in order to be properly interpreted, many other factors have to be taken into consideration.

The heart rate is under the influence of two sets of nerves. The sympathetic nervous system increases the rate, whilst the parasympathetic nervous system decreases it. The latter develops later in fetal life, which is why premature infants have a higher intrinsic rate. This falls to the 'mature' range at about 30 weeks' gestation.

The sympathetic and parasympathetic nervous systems are not balanced in their opposing effects, so the heart rate fluctuates. Beat-to-beat variability (i.e. the continual change in rate) is too fast to be picked up on a CTG (as 140 beats would have to be fitted into a 1 cm space); instead it is the fluctuating baseline that is recorded. This is 'baseline variability', or simply 'variability' or 'reactivity'.

## BASELINE RATE

This is normally 120–160 beats per minute (bpm), although in a healthy term infant it may be 110 bpm. Here are some of the causes of a slow rate (bradycardia, Figure 1) and a fast rate (tachycardia, Figure 2).

| **Bradycardia** | **Tachycardia** |
|---|---|
| Maturity | Prematurity |
| Fetal compromise | Fetal compromise |
| Fall in blood pressure | Causes of maternal tachycardia |
| —some antihypertensive drugs | —tocolytics, e.g. salbutamol |

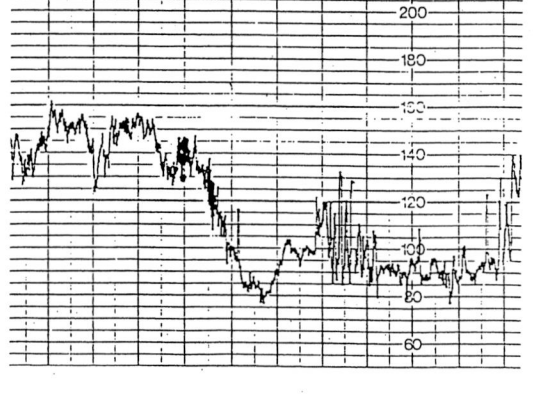

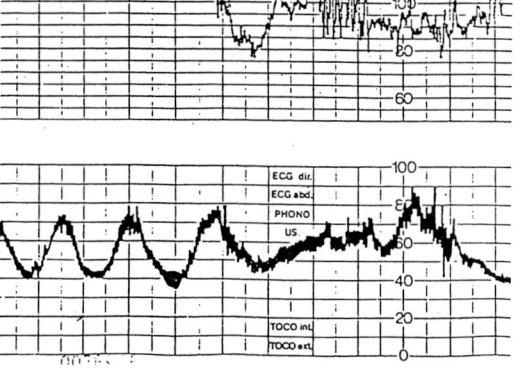

**Fig. 1** Bradycardia, as seen after an epidural top-up or a hypertonic contraction

—epidural top-up      —pyrexia
—supine hypotension    —hydrallazine
                          —phenothiazines sometimes
Sedation, e.g. pethidine   Fetal anaemia
After amniotomy        (also causes sinusoidal trace)
Head rotation           Fetal cardiac arrhythmias
Congenital heart block

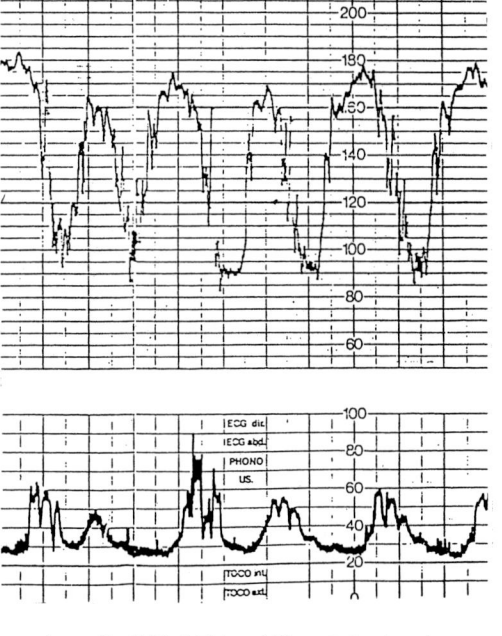

**Fig. 2** Baseline tachycardia (170–180 bpm). Type 2 decelerations

A steady bradycardia is less worrying than a sudden fall in rate.

## BASELINE VARIABILITY
This gives the best indication of fetal well-being, provided that an appropriate time span is monitored. Reduced variability is usually normal and occurs during periods of fetal inactivity or 'rest', but

prolonged episodes suggest chronic hypoxia and fetal compromise. The average time that a fetus spends in the resting state is 20 minutes, although it may be as long as 40 minutes both antenatally and during labour. Variability is greatest at night and lowest between 06:00 and 12:00. The average full cycle of rest–activity–rest is 90 minutes.

Two examples of rest–activity cycles are shown on pages 4–5, the first before (Figure 3) and the second during labour (Figure 4).

When interpreting a CTG with reduced variability, it is therefore important to remember that one might be observing a rest period, and so the tracing should be continued until a period of activity is seen.

A rest, or sleep, pattern may also be seen after administration of sedatives, some analgesics and hypotensive drugs. If a reduction of variability is seen over a prolonged period of time and if there are decelerations or the presence of meconium, fetal compromise should be suspected and either fetal blood sampling performed or delivery expedited, whichever is the most appropriate.

Baseline variability is classified as:

Silent    =  0–5 bpm
Reduced =  6–10 bpm
Normal  =  10–25 bpm
Saltatory =  >25 bpm

A sinusoidal trace, sometimes seen in fetal anaemia, oscillates 2–5 times per minute, with no short-term variability and with an amplitude of 5–10 bpm (but sometimes up to 60 bpm, which worsens the prognosis). An example has not been included as there is controversy regarding both its diagnosis and implications. Fetal anaemia may also result in a 'flat' trace, with greatly reduced variability, or in a baseline tachycardia.

## ACCELERATIONS (Figure 5)

Accelerations are an increase of at least 15 bpm for 15 seconds, and should occur at least twice in a 20-minute period, during the activity part of the cycle, for the trace to be classified as reactive. If very reactive, the trace may give the appearance of a baseline tachycardia with decelerations, so look for a more stable period to assess the baseline rate. Towards the end of pregnancy, both the amplitude and frequency of accelerations increase. Before 28 weeks there are usually only two accelerations per hour, this increases to about 12 at 34 weeks and sometimes 18 at term.

It is difficult to quantify the normal range of reactivity within the population and some fetuses may exhibit prolonged inactivity and yet be entirely healthy. Sometimes other parameters may suggest fetal well-being, but if the CTG is used alone it is always best to err on the side of caution.

## DECELERATIONS
### Artefactual

These are rapid vertical lines, often due to momentary loss of contact during maternal movement, and do not represent a change in fetal rate.

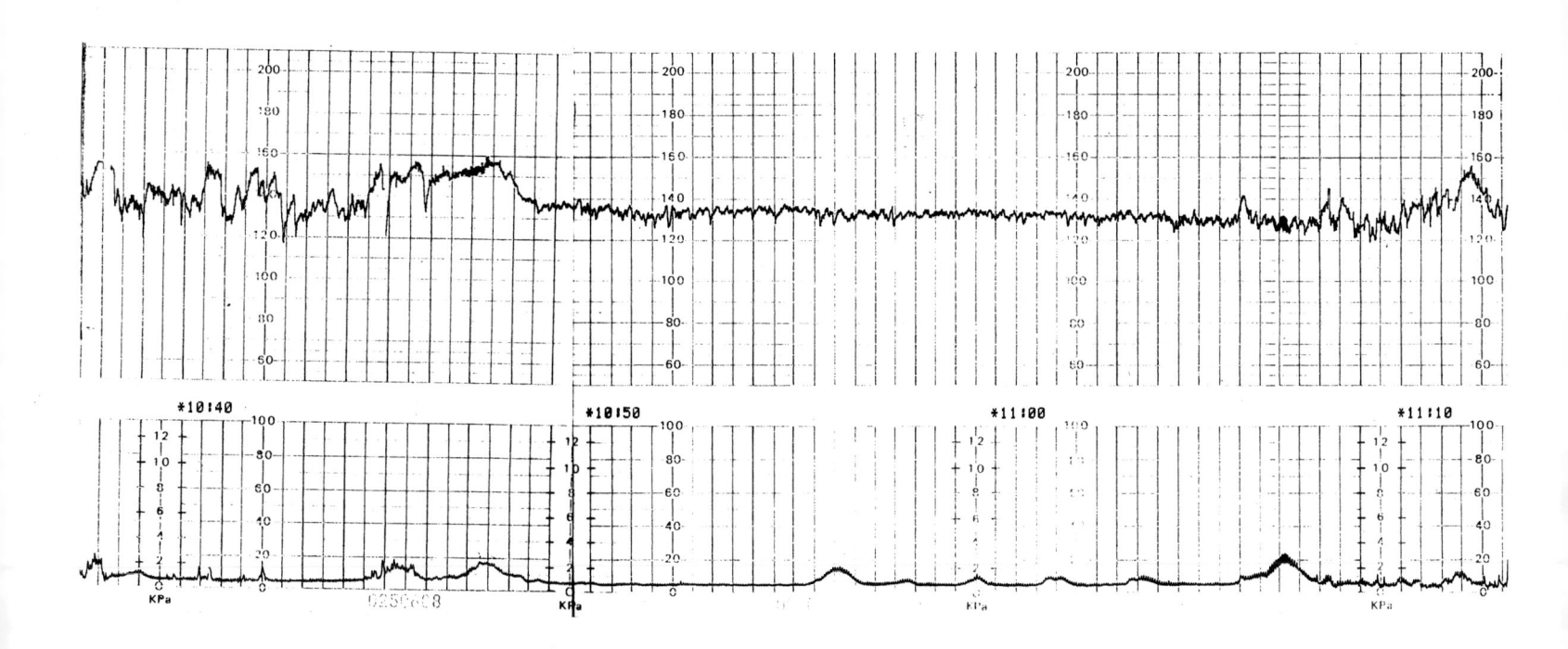

**Fig. 3** Rest–activity cycling antenatally

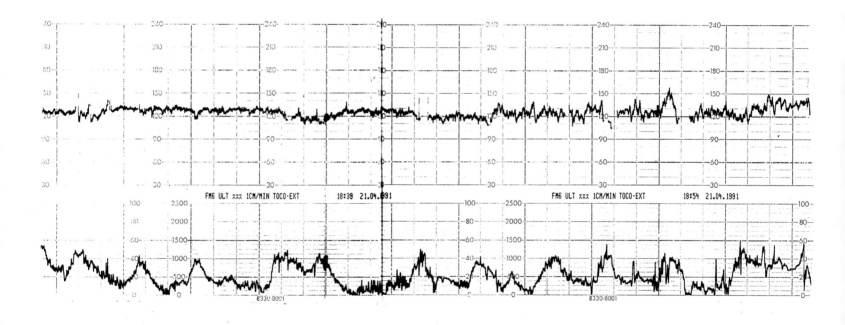

FM6 ULT ××× 1CM/MIN TOCO-EXT    18:39 21.04.891

FM6 ULT ××× 1CM/MIN TOCO-EXT    18:54 21.04.1991

8330-8001

8330-8001

**Fig. 4** Rest–activity cycling in labour

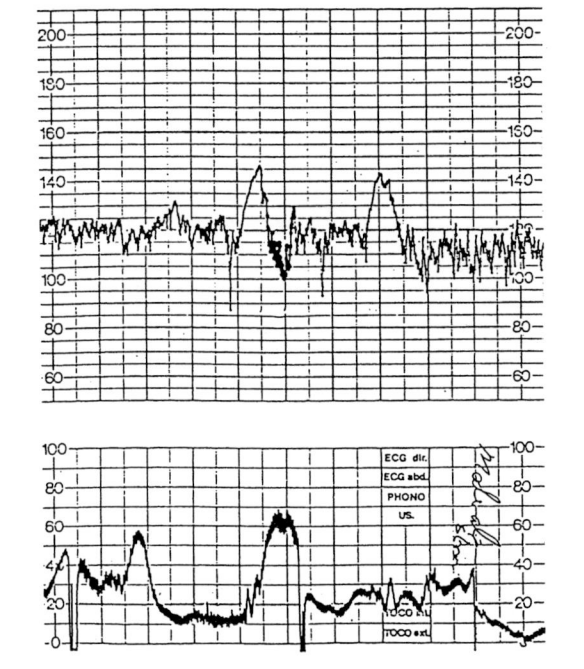

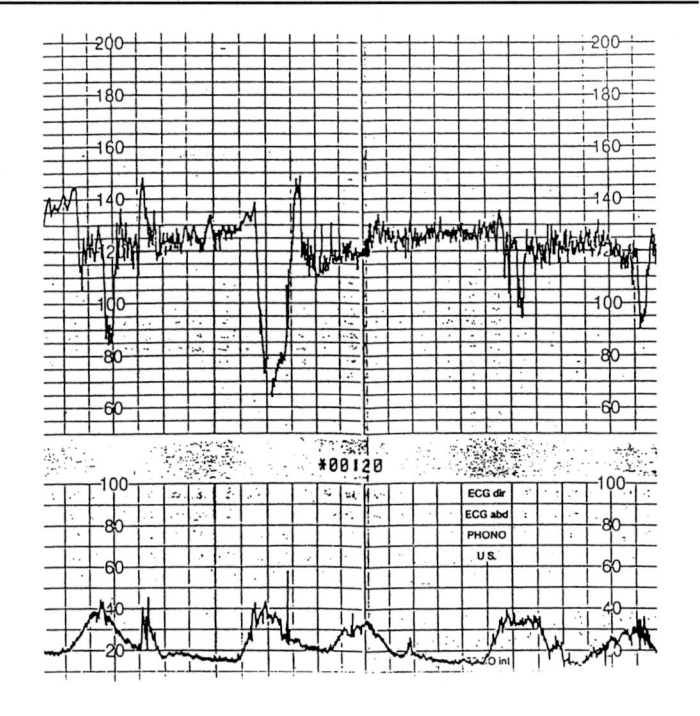

**Fig. 5** Reactive trace with accelerations. Note baseline 110–120 bpm (normal in some mature babies)

**Fig. 6** Reactive trace with Type 1 decelerations and accelerations

### Early (Type 1, synchronous) (Figure 6)
Their nadir coincides with a uterine contraction and recovery is rapid. They are usually due to head compression and are rarely deeper than 40 bpm and do not suggest fetal compromise. If they are worsening, consider cephalopelvic disproportion (CPD).

### Late (Type 2, asynchronous) (Figure 7)
These occur in between contractions. Decelerations are also so named when a Type 1 deceleration recovers slowly, after the contraction has worn off. The late deceleration suggests asphyxia due to reduced placental oxygenation, especially if there is an abnormal

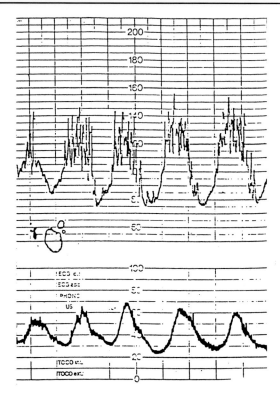

**Fig. 7** Type 2 decelerations

rate or change in baseline with no accelerations, reduced variability, passage of meconium or a slow recovery. Other bad signs are an exaggerated acceleration after the deceleration or a 'W'-shaped deceleration (i.e. worsening again before it recovers). A prolonged deceleration with no variability within is an ominous sign.

**Variable (Figure 8)**
These are a combination of Type 1 and 2 with variable shape and timing. They may be due to cord compression, when the cord may be twisted around the fetal neck or a limb, knotted or prolapsed. Their significance depends on other factors; that is, they are acceptable if there is a good rate and variability, but worrying if there are the features described for Type 2 decelerations.

Other causes of decelerations include:

—Vaginal examination
—Hypertonic contractions
   —sometimes due to oxytocin (Syntocinon) or prostaglandins
—Head rotation or rapid descent
—Spontaneous membrane rupture or amniotomy
—Supine hypotension (lying in the dorsal position)
—Rapid drop in blood pressure
   —epidural top-ups
   —placental abruption
   —antihypertensive injections
—Sometimes narcotics

**SECOND STAGE**
In the second stage it is normal to see deeper decelerations, usually Type 1. It is important that they return to their previous baseline. Delivery should be expedited if the baseline is falling or if the

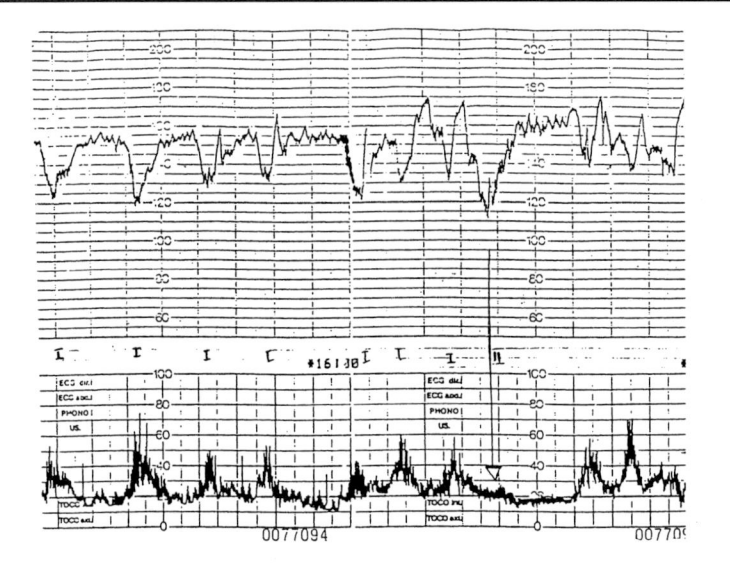

**Fig. 8** Variable decelerations of mostly Type 1; reactive baseline 150–160 bpm; some accelerations; fetus unlikely to be badly compromised

decelerations are late, prolonged and associated with reduced variability.

## QUALITY OF THE CARDIOTOCOGRAPH

The quality of the CTG is dependent upon the sophistication of the technology and the maintenance of the machine. Older models have greater mechanical artefact which can be mistaken for fetal reactivity!

A fetal scalp electrode provides a better quality recording than an external transducer and is particularly useful when an epidural is being used, as alterations in the position of the mother on the bed may cause loss of contact with an external transducer.

Interpretation of the CTG is not always easy. Many factors other than just the heart rate need to be considered, and of course the progress of labour is also important. Sometimes rapid descent and rotation of the head with quick cervical dilatation can result in worrying decelerations and then a swift spontaneous delivery of a normal baby.

Clear liquor is a good sign, but absence of liquor does not exclude meconium, which may be dammed up behind a head that is being 'jammed' into the pelvis. To say for certain that the fetus is distressed, a sample of fetal scalp blood should be taken to assess the degree of acidosis and hypoxia—this was unfortunately not available to us on our labour ward, and so the CTG alone was heavily relied upon. In the last three cases, we provide examples of how fetal blood sampling may be employed.

There follows a series of CTGs taken from women in labour. They are not continuous but represent several short periods during each labour, thus showing how things can change. Before each set of traces is a brief maternal history. After the traces a copy of the partogram is included in some cases, then a record of the outcome and our intepretation of and comments on the traces.

It is suggested that you read the history then write your own comments about each trace, study the partogram and then look at our summary of the outcome and interpretation of the CTGs.

For each trace look at the baseline rate and variability, nature of the trace (i.e. accelerations, decelerations...) and uterine activity. Clues can be taken from comments written on the trace. As CTG intepretation is often subjective our opinions may not always be the same as everyone else's, but we have tried to be as objective as possible.

Doctors' signatures on CTGs have been masked.

# CASE 1

21-year Somalian refugee

G2 P0 + 1 (1988 TOP at
10 weeks)
No past history
Circumcised

LMP 28.8.89—EDD 5.6.90
           —EDD by scan
             23.6.90

Booked 16 weeks
Shared care

28.6.90 40+ weeks

03:40    Admitted with contractions since 23:00
          Cephalic presentation
          Left occipito-transverse (LOT) position
          Head 2/5 palpable abdominally
          Cervix 3 cm dilated
          Membranes bulging
          Weak contractions only

08:00    6 cm
          Amniotomy, LOT
          Fetal scalp electrode eventually applied
          after decelerations

11:30    Fully dilated

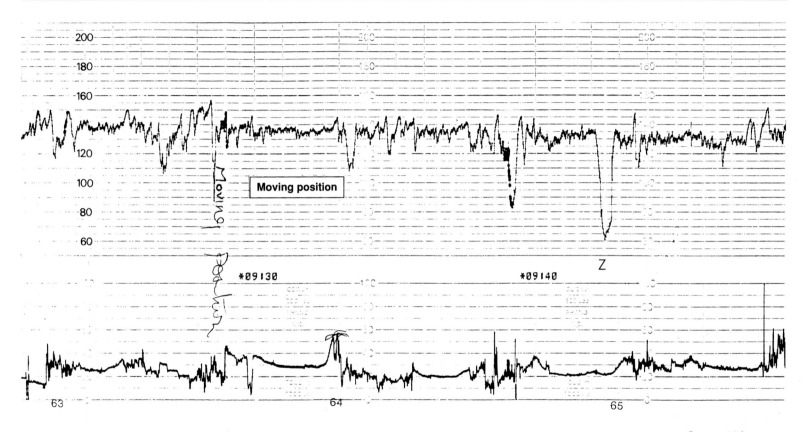

Moving position

*09130   *09140   Z

See page 16 for outcome

# 1.2

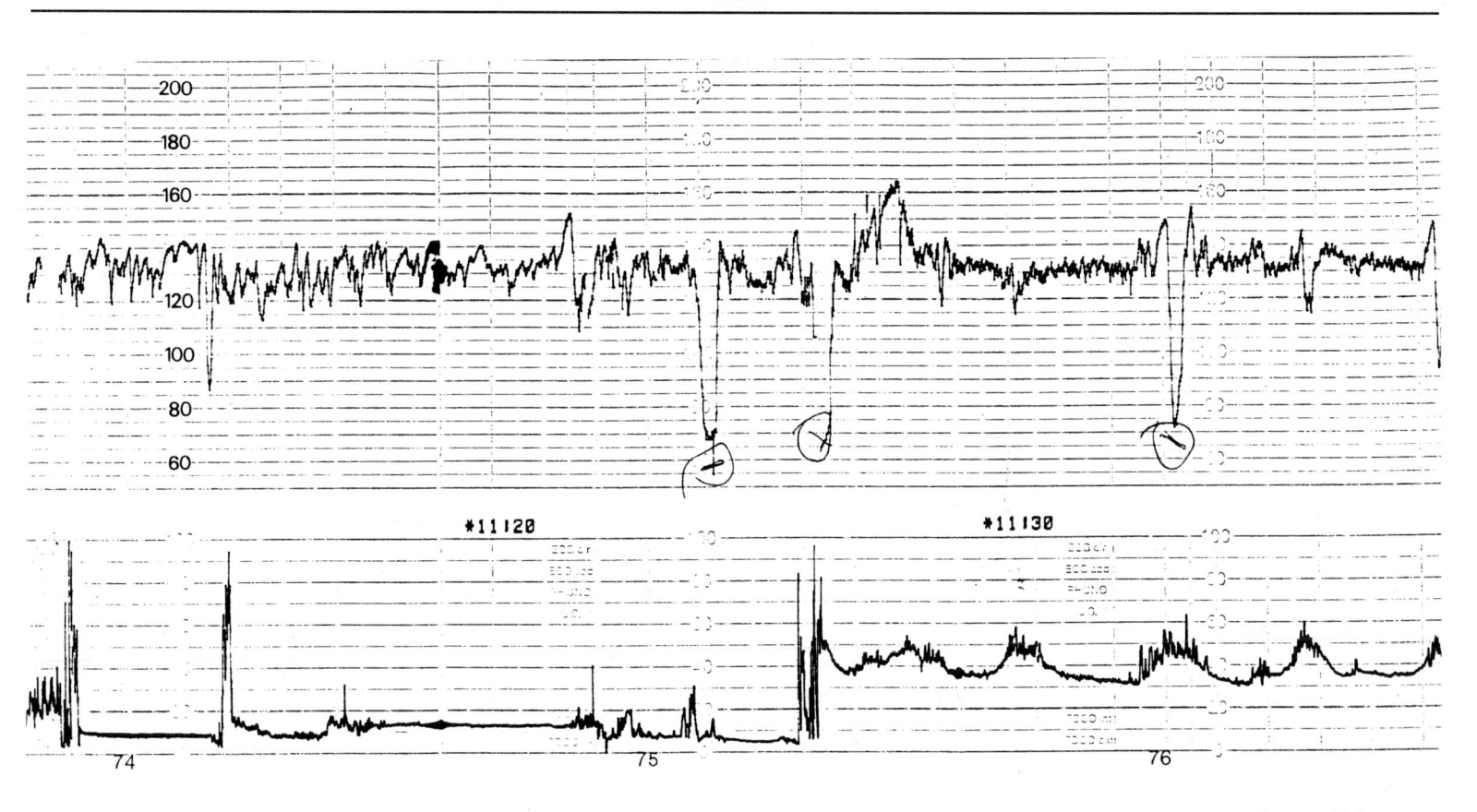

*See page 16 for outcome*

# 1.3

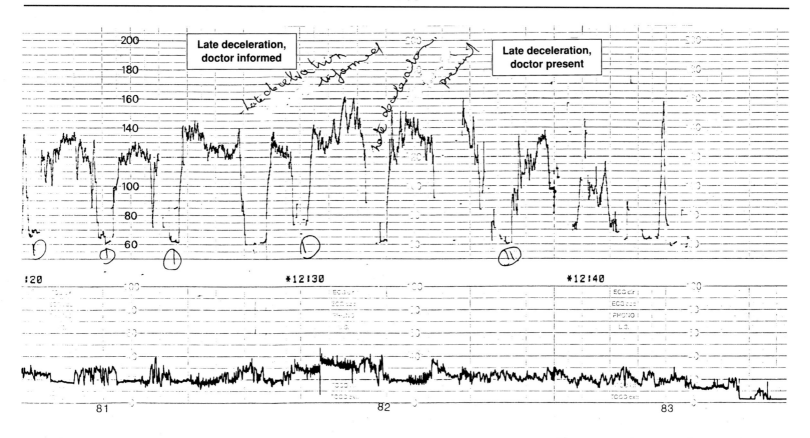

See page 16 for outcome

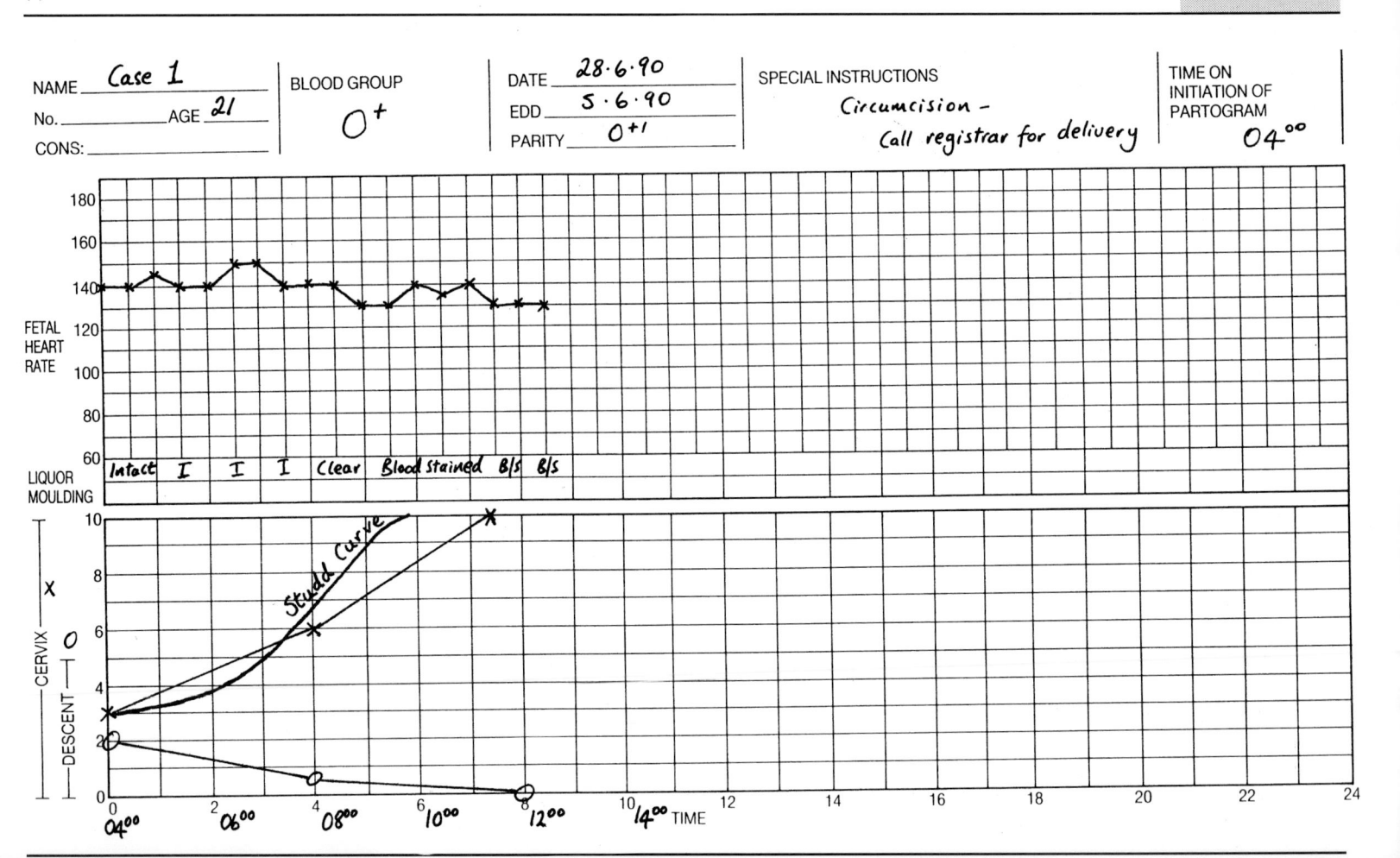

NAME _Case 1_

No. _____ AGE _21_

CONS: _____

BLOOD GROUP

$O^+$

DATE _28.6.90_

EDD _5.6.90_

PARITY _0+1_

SPECIAL INSTRUCTIONS

_Circumcision –_

_Call registrar for delivery_

TIME ON
INITIATION OF
PARTOGRAM

_04⁰⁰_

FETAL
HEART
RATE

180
160
140
120
100
80
60

LIQUOR
MOULDING

| Intact | I | I | I | Clear | Blood Stained | B/S | B/S |

CERVIX X 0
DESCENT

Studd Curve

10
8
6
4
2
0

0
04⁰⁰   2 06⁰⁰   4 08⁰⁰   6 10⁰⁰   8 12⁰⁰   10 14⁰⁰ TIME   12   14   16   18   20   22   24

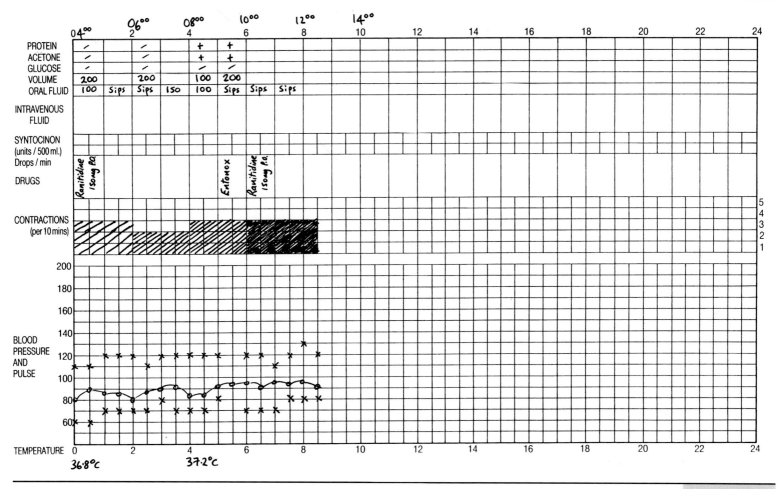

# Outcome

12:45   Left occipito-anterior (LOA), spontaneous delivery
Elective right mediolateral episiotomy performed because of circumcision
3.6 kg male
Apgars 5/1 (1 minute) 9/5 (5 minutes)
Cord twice around neck

**1.1**
A healthy reactive trace with Type 1 decelerations and some accelerations. Baseline 140 bpm. Z may be a Type 2 deceleration, but it is short-lived and has an acceleration soon after. We would not worry about this.

**1.2**
This is still very reactive, with accelerations and Type 1 decelerations.

**1.3**
The baseline is reactive; Type 1 decelerations are broader and the baseline is dropping. This is consistent with an advancing head and cord around the neck. As the fetus was obviously advancing and about to deliver intervention was not necessary.

When the baseline starts to fall in the second stage one should aim for delivery within 10–15 minutes (see Case 2).

# Clinical points

## PAPER SPEED

Remember the paper speed is 1 cm/minute, so 2 small squares = 1 minute; and 10 minutes is 20 squares, or the distance between each column of numbers.

## CIRCUMCISION

Some communities still perform circumcision on young girls. This horrific procedure is painful, damaging and may result in severe haemorrhage and infection. It is thus vital to reassure the mother, who is likely to be very frightened, that adequate analgesia will be provided during parturition. It is usually necessary to perform an episiotomy and if there is severe scarring this may need to be divided anteriorly.

## THE PARTOGRAM: 1

The partogram provides a graphical record not only of progress in labour, but also of changes in fetal and maternal condition and of all drugs and intravenous fluids that have been administered. In such a condensed form all necessary information can be seen at a glance.

Short-term variations in fetal heart rate are monitored by the CTG, whilst longer term changes in baseline rate can be viewed more easily on the partogram. This may then be compared with the maternal heart rate, so if both are rising and the mother is pyrexial you have identified the probable cause of the fetal tachycardia.

The partogram should be commenced when labour starts. If a woman is admitted in established labour it is still advisable to detail all observations, as one cannot easily predict what may still happen!

The first page of the partogram also depicts the progressive dilatation of the cervix together with the descent of the fetal head. The latter is more reliably assessed by abdominal, rather than vaginal, examination (see Case 22). The expected rate of cervical dilatation can be plotted with a Studd stencil (Rocket of London Ltd, Imperial Way, Watford). In the active phase of labour, cervimetric progress is similar in primigravidae and multiparous women. If the rate of progress strays to the right of the drawn line by 2 hours or more you should look for signs of dysfunctional uterine activity and/or cephalopelvic disproportion. Appropriate action must then be taken; for example, augmenting labour with oxytocin or performing a caesarean section. Some partograms have a pre-drawn 'alert line' and 'action line'.

*Cross references:* **The partogram** *pages 23, 85* **The falling baseline** *page 23* **The fetal scalp electrode** *page 151*

CASE 1

# CASE 2

21-year single, home help

Primigravida
No past history

LMP 13.4.89—EDD 20.1.90

Booked at 16 weeks
Shared care
Uneventful pregnancy

28.1.90 41+ weeks

| | |
|---|---|
| 09:30 | Admitted with spontaneous rupture of membranes (SROM)<br>High head, 4/5 palpable<br>Left occipito-transverse position<br>Cervix closed<br>Clear liquor |
| 22:45 | Pethidine given<br>1 cm dilated |
| 02:45 | 4 cm<br>Fetal scalp electrode applied |
| 03:15 | 5 cm |
| 03:45 | Fully dilated |

# 2.1

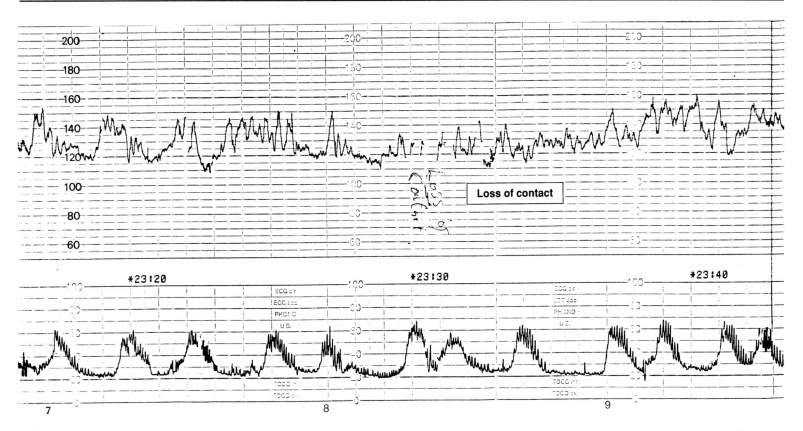

**Loss of contact**

*23:20  *23:30  *23:40

ECG dir
ECG abd
PHONO
U.S.

TOCO int
TOCO ext

7    8    9

*See page 22 for outcome*

**CASE 2**

## 2.2

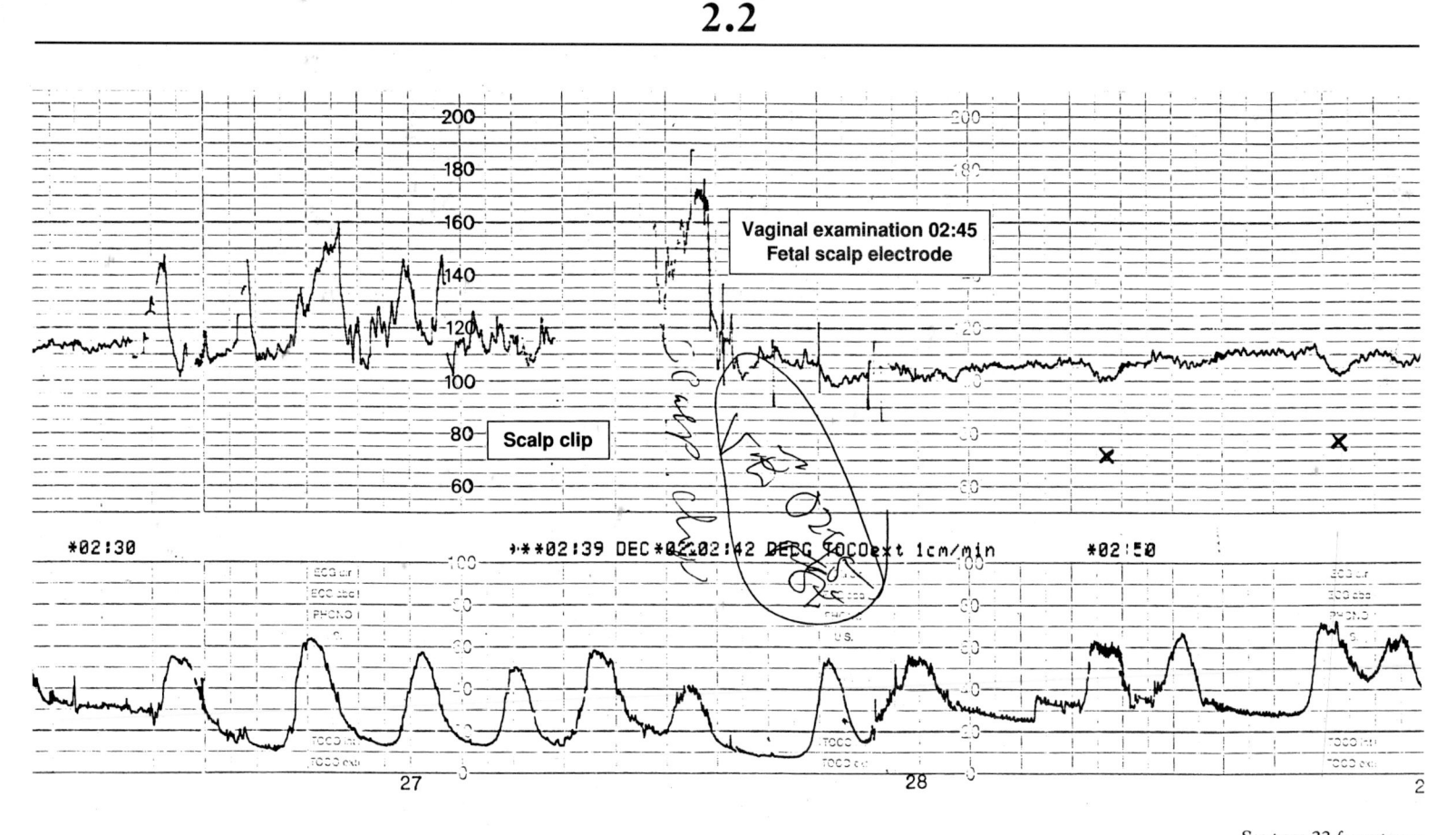

Vaginal examination 02:45
Fetal scalp electrode

Scalp clip

See page 22 for outcome

# 2.3

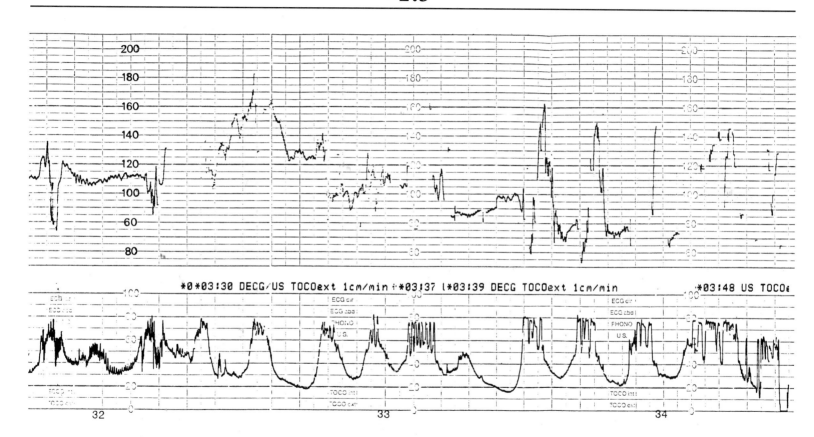

*0*03:30 DECG/US TOCOext 1cm/min *03:37 (*03:39 DECG TOCOext 1cm/min          *03:48 US TOCO

See page 22 for outcome

**CASE 2**

# Outcome

03:55   Spontaneous delivery
        4.45 kg female
        Apgars 6/1 9/5

No partogram was kept.

**2.1**
Good variability with accelerations from a baseline of 120 bpm. There is some 'coupling' of the contractions, with one following another without a period of uterine relaxation. This is a sign of dysfunctional uterine activity.

**2.2**
The baseline has dropped a little and a fetal scalp electrode is applied; there are large accelerations and then a sleep pattern with shallow Type 1 decelerations (X), suggesting the need for continuous monitoring. Hypoxia is unlikely.

The contractions are still not completely regular.

**2.3**
The second stage was only 15–20 minutes. The large swings in heart rate suggest fetal decompensation and a further drop in baseline to 80–90 bpm is worrying if delivery is not imminent. As mentioned previously, a falling baseline in the second stage indicates that the baby needs to be delivered. In this case this was occurring spontaneously and intervention was not required, but we would not have been happy to see this type of trace continue for any longer.

# Clinical points

## FALLING BASELINE

In the second stage of labour a steady baseline of normal rate gives the best prognosis. Decelerations that are becoming more pronounced with each successive contraction should not be allowed to persist for more than 15–20 minutes, and if they have a variable pattern one should suspect cord compression. If the baseline rate falls one should aim for delivery within 15 minutes, although a bradycardia of 100 bpm or less warrants delivery in 5 minutes.

It is important to be aware of changes in baseline rate, so that a tachycardia with decelerations is not mistaken for a bradycadia with accelerations.

## THE PARTOGRAM: 2

On the second page of the partogram details are recorded of the maternal condition and of the drugs and fluids given. The strength of the contractions, as well as their frequency, may be symbolized by the density of cross-hatches in the boxes. If blood pressure and pulse rise and the contractions are getting stronger, consider analgesia rather than antihypertensives (provided there is no underlying worry about hypertension).

Fluid balance in labour is very important. The volume of all urine voided should be recorded along with a urinalysis of each specimen. Dehydration is depicted by more concentrated urine (rising specific gravity) and ketonuria. This should be corrected by either oral or intravenous rehydration, depending upon the condition of the mother.

Dehydration results in a more uncomfortable labour. If there is oliguria it is important to exclude hypovolaemic shock and renal disorders, all of which should be suggested by other aspects of the history and examination.

Proteinuria is almost an invariable finding during labour and is usually secondary to contamination. If there is concern about either proteinuric hypertension or a urinary tract infection a catheter should be passed to obtain a 'clean' specimen of urine. In so doing you should be scrupulous about aseptic technique, as during labour there is a high risk of introducing infection. Many obstetricians recommend a postpartum urine microscopy for all women who are catheterized in labour, whatever the reason.

*Cross references:* **The partogram** *pages 17, 85* **The fetal scalp electrode** *page 151* **Intravenous fluids** *pages 175, 176*

# CASE 3

20-year bank clerk

Primigravida

1987 left ovarian cystectomy

LMP 21.9.89—EDD 28.6.90

Booked at 15 weeks
Shared care

Uneventful pregnancy

25.6.90 39+ weeks

| | |
|---|---|
| 23:50 | Admitted contracting<br>Cephalic presentation<br>Head 2/5 palpable per abdomen<br>Right occipito-posterior (ROP) position<br>Cervix 3 cm dilated<br>Spontaneous rupture of membranes, clear liquor |
| 03:45 | 3 cm<br>Pethidine given |
| 05:45 | 3–4 cm<br>Occipito-posterior position |
| 08:10 | 4 cm, meconium<br>Epidural then oxytocin |
| 11:55 | 6 cm |
| 16:00 | Fully dilated<br>ROP position<br>Temperature 38.2°C |

# 3.1

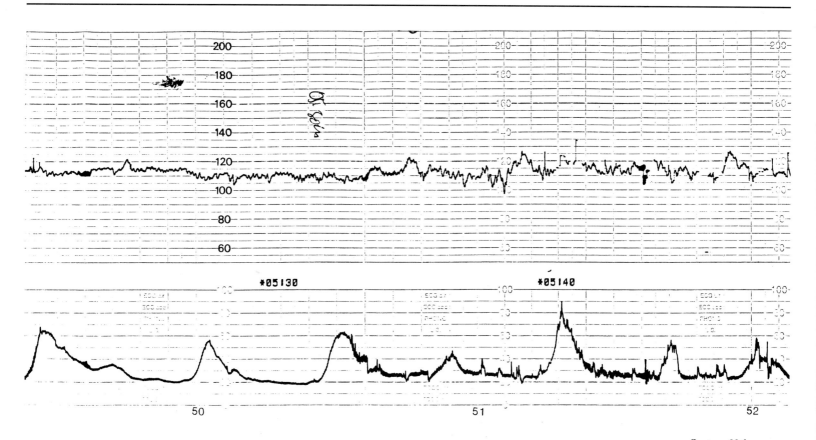

*See page 32 for outcome*

# 3.2

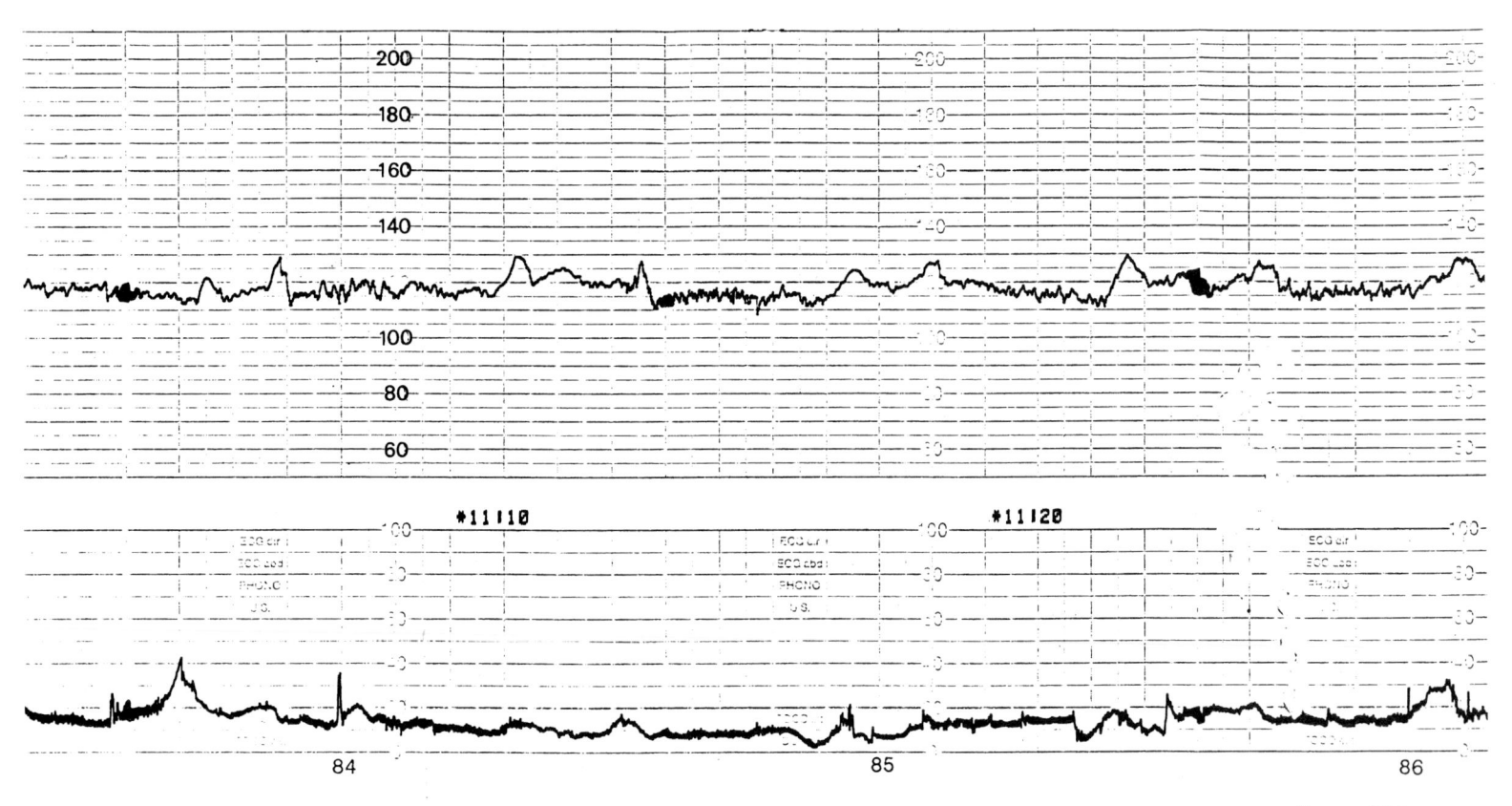

*See page 32 for outcome*

# 3.3

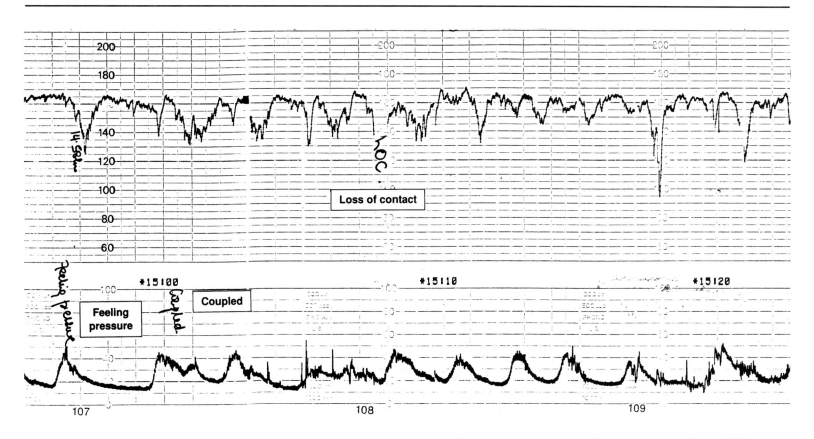

*See page 32 for outcome*

# 3.4

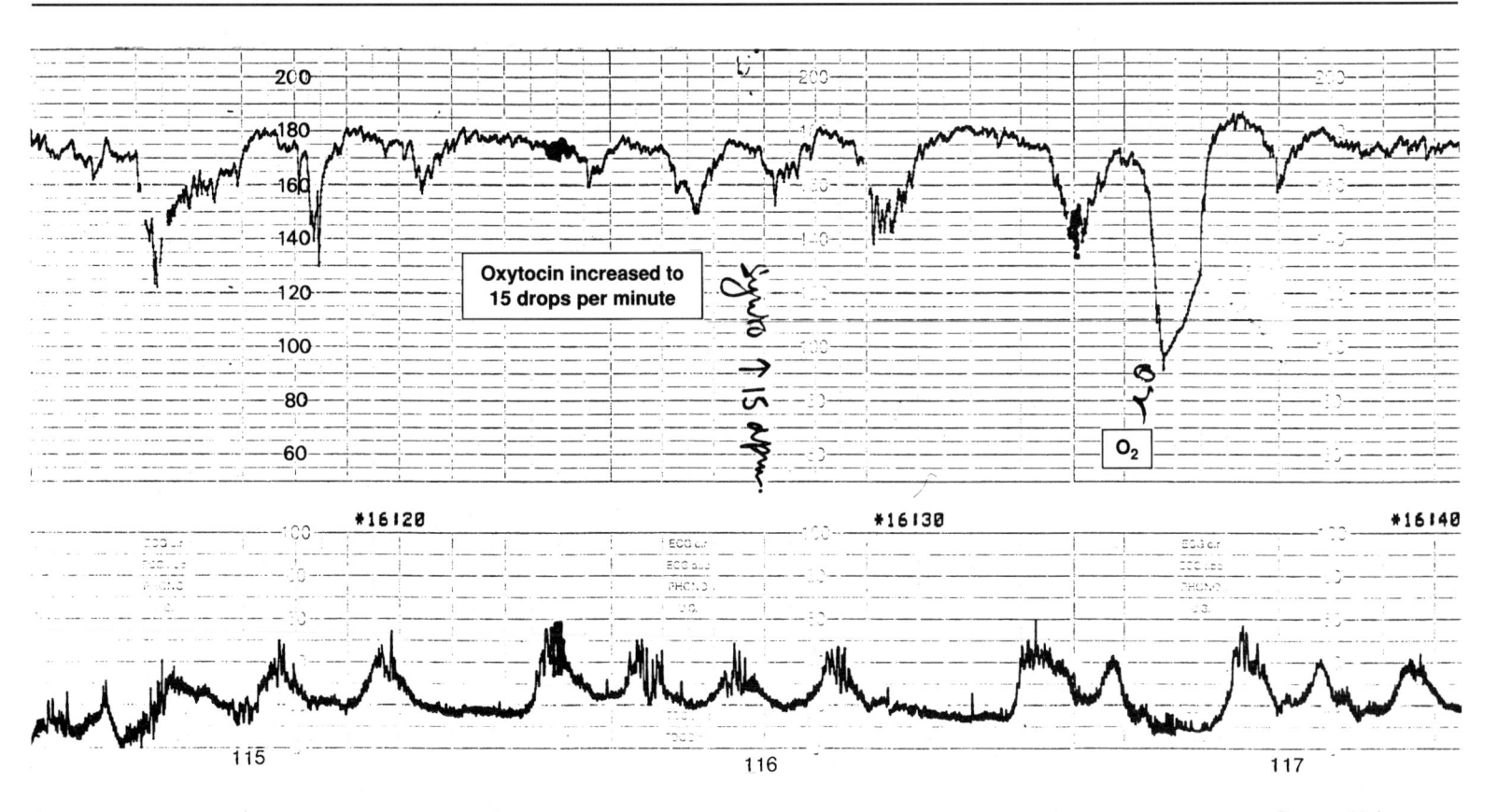

**Oxytocin increased to 15 drops per minute**

O₂

*See page 32 for outcome*

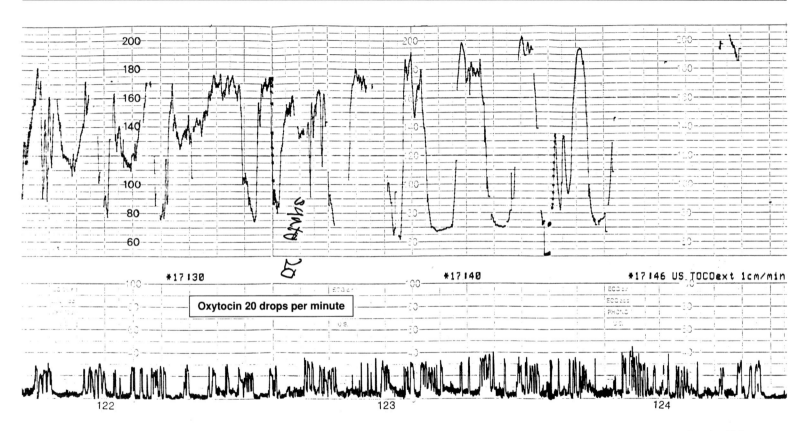

Oxytocin 20 drops per minute

*17130  *17140  *17146 US TOCOext 1cm/min

122  123  124

*See page 32 for outcome*

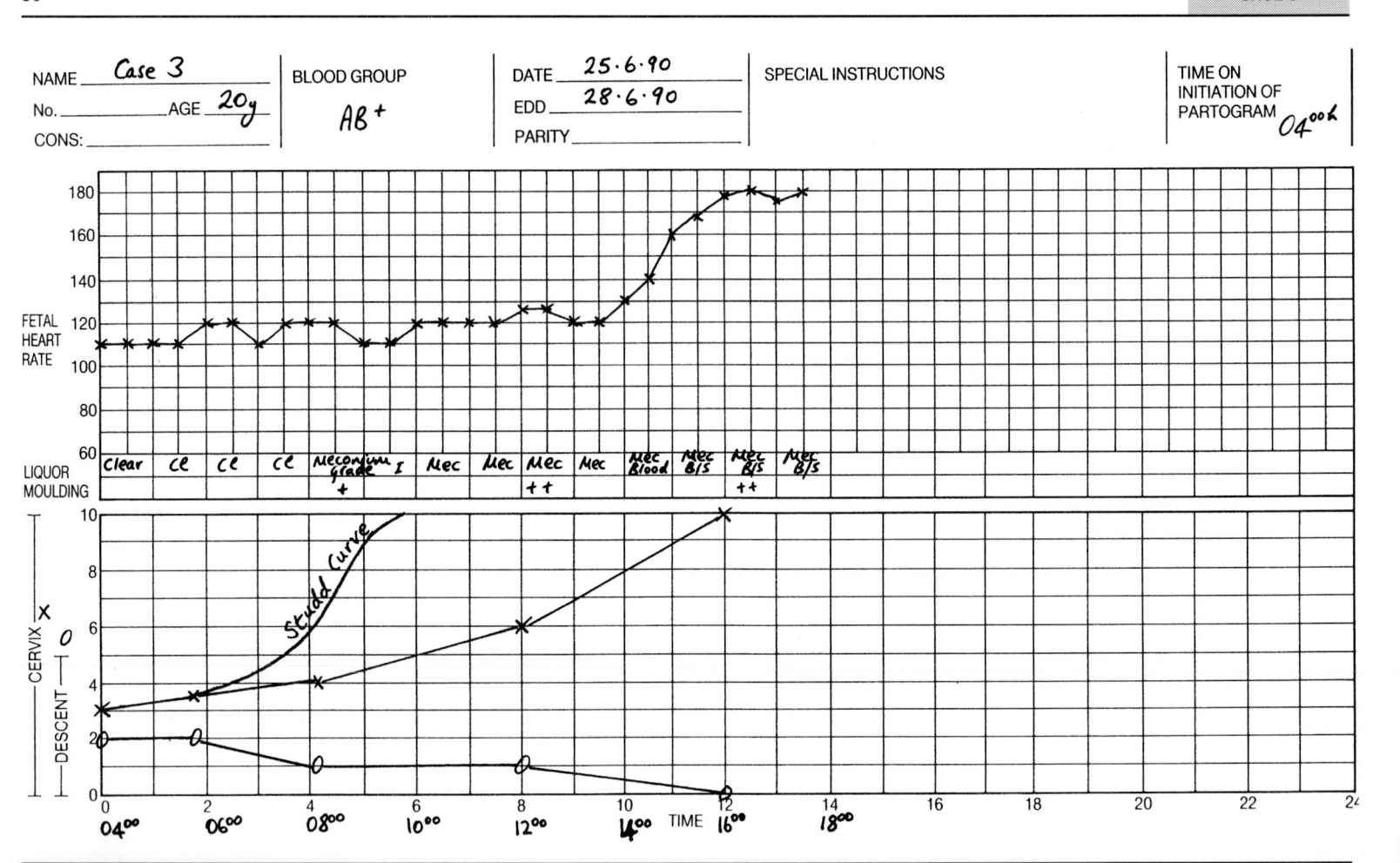

NAME __Case 3__

No. _____ AGE __20y__

CONS: _____

BLOOD GROUP

__AB+__

DATE __25·6·90__

EDD __28·6·90__

PARITY _____

SPECIAL INSTRUCTIONS

TIME ON INITIATION OF PARTOGRAM __04⁰⁰ʰ__

FETAL HEART RATE

| LIQUOR MOULDING | Clear | Cl | Cl | Cl | Meconium grade I + | Mec | Mec | Mec ++ | Mec | Mec Blood | Mec B/S | Mec B/S ++ | Mec B/S |

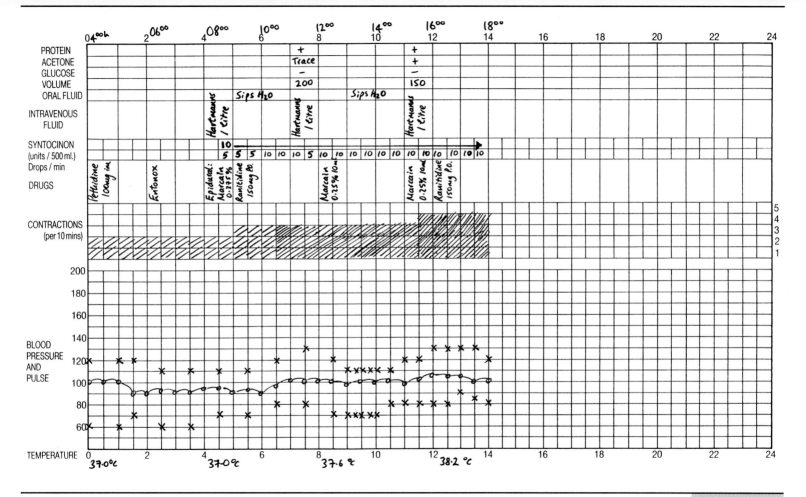

# Outcome

17:25 Pushing commenced
17:53 Spontaneous delivery
2.85 kg female
Apgars 5/1 7/5 9/10
Intubated, oxygen given

**3.1**
Baseline 110 bpm; initially sleep pattern—possibly an effect of the pethidine; then good variability with accelerations. A baseline of 110 in a term infant is *not* classified as significant bradycardia, although a change in baseline may be significant.

**3.2**
Several hours later the baseline has risen slightly; the variability is only 5 bpm, but there are accelerations. Oxytocin was started for slow progress—perhaps a little late.

**3.3**
The baseline has risen to 160 bpm. Maternal temperature is 37.6°C; this could be secondary to the epidural or as a result of intrauterine infection. There are variable decelerations, mostly Type 2 with quick recovery and good variability. If available, fetal blood sampling should be performed now, although there is unlikely to be severe fetal compromise.

**3.4**
The baseline has risen further and the Type 2 decelerations are broader. The patient is fully dilated and so it is time to think about delivery fairly soon.

**3.5**
The mother was left perhaps longer than we would like. Deeper decelerations are often seen in the second stage, but on top of the compromise already seen the baby was born flat and requiring resuscitation.

This woman had a long labour due to an occipito-posterior position. Perhaps she should have had an epidural and augmentation earlier. The liquor was initially clear, but became meconium-stained.

# Clinical points

## EPIDURAL PYREXIA

When an epidural is used the maternal temperature commonly rises by about 0.5° C for every 6 hours in labour. This is due mainly to a paralysis of the lumbosacral parasympathetic nerves, which prevents the sweating that dissipates about 80 % of body heat. The resultant fetal pyrexia may lead to a fetal tachycardia and acidosis. It is therefore important to fan the mother and keep her well hydrated.

Chorioamnionitis may still occur in the presence of an epidural and this important cause of a pyrexia should not be forgotten.

## MECONIUM: 1

Meconium can be graded:

I:   light-coloured, staining predominantly clear liquor
II:  between I and II
III: thick, 'pea soup', with no liquor

It is the relative amount of liquor diluting the meconium that is important. Grade III therefore carries the worst prognosis as it reflects a reduction in liquor volume. Meconium is associated with an increased chance of intrapartum stillbirth, neonatal morbidity and death. It will usually have been passed prior to the onset of labour and it denotes antenatal compromise, such as impaired placental function, and hence an increased chance of hypoxia in labour. The presence of Grade III meconium warrants fetal blood sampling, if available.

The absence of visible liquor may mean that meconium is damming up behind the fetal head. So if there is no liquor to be seen it is possible gently to pass a fine catheter (e.g. infant feeding tube) up beside the fetal head, allowing liquor ± meconium to descend. This procedure is only safe if the placental site is known—and avoided!

Cross references:   **Epidurals**  *pages 40, 99*   **Meconium**  *page 118*

# CASE 4

25-year Jamaican, single,
auxillary nurse

Primigravida
No past history

EDD 11.5.90

Booked 12 weeks
Uneventful pregnancy

| | |
|---|---|
| 8.5.90 | 39+ weeks |
| 06:30 | 'Show' and contractions |
| | Cephalic presentation |
| | Right occipito-transverse (ROT) position |
| | Head 3–4/5 palpable |
| | Cervix 2 cm dilated |
| | Intact membranes |
| 09:15 | 3 cm |
| | Amniotomy, clear liquor |
| 10:55 | Epidural |
| | Fall in blood pressure, ephedrine given |
| 11:20 | 4 cm |
| | ROT, head still high |

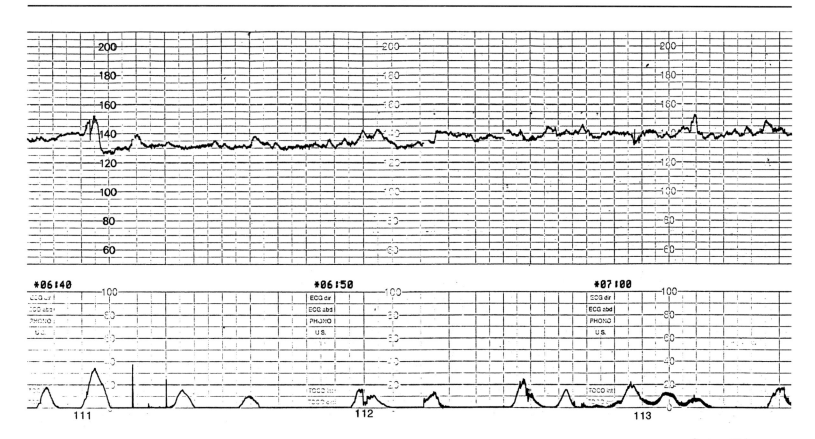

*See page 39 for outcome*

# 4.2

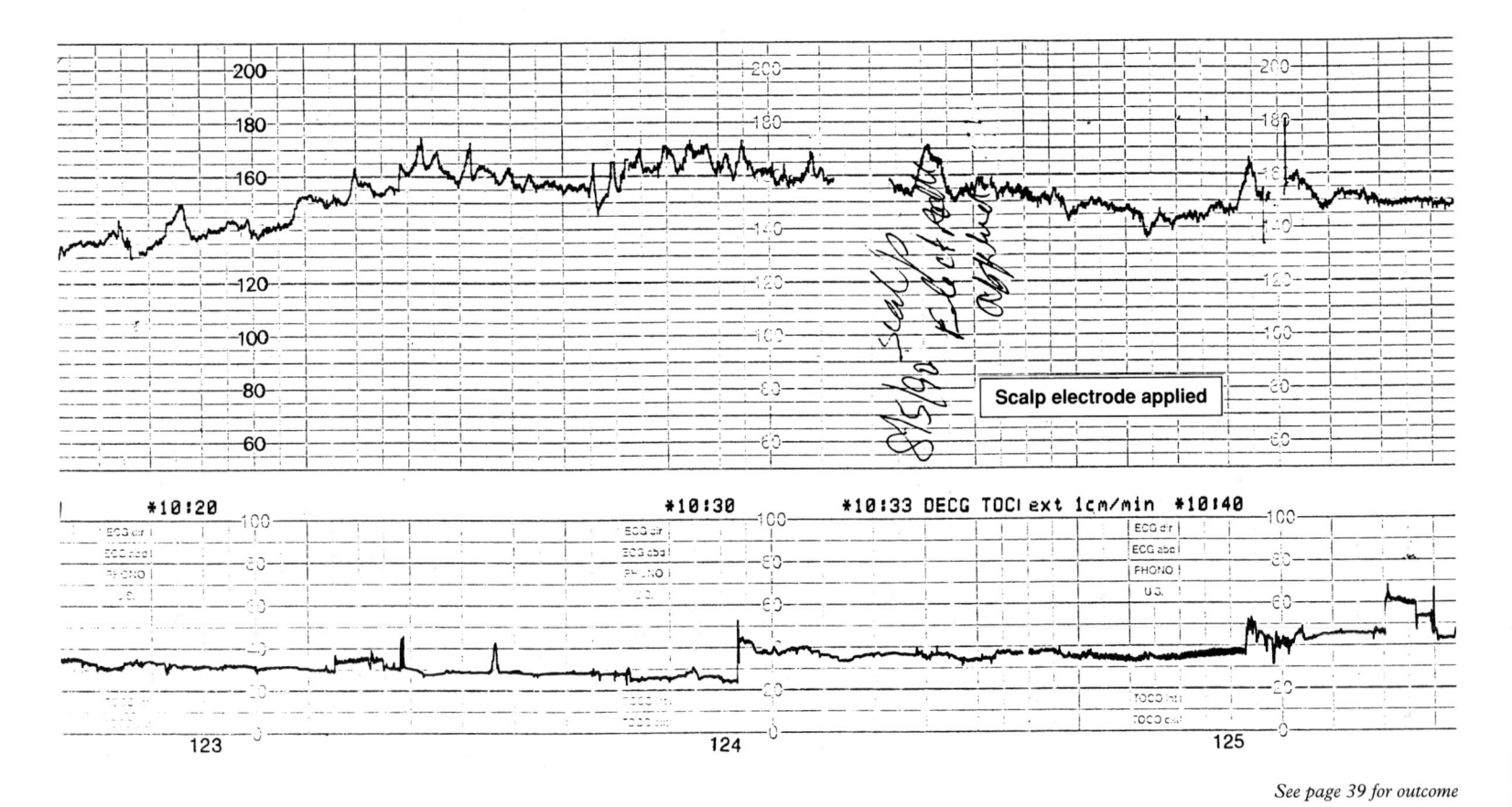

Scalp electrode applied

*10:20    *10:30    *10:33 DECG TOCI ext 1cm/min    *10:40

123    124    125

*See page 39 for outcome*

# 4.3

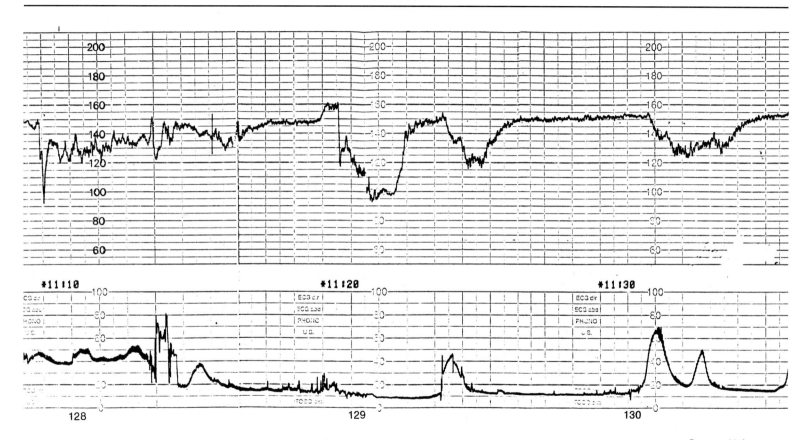

*See page 39 for outcome*

**CASE 4**

# 4.4

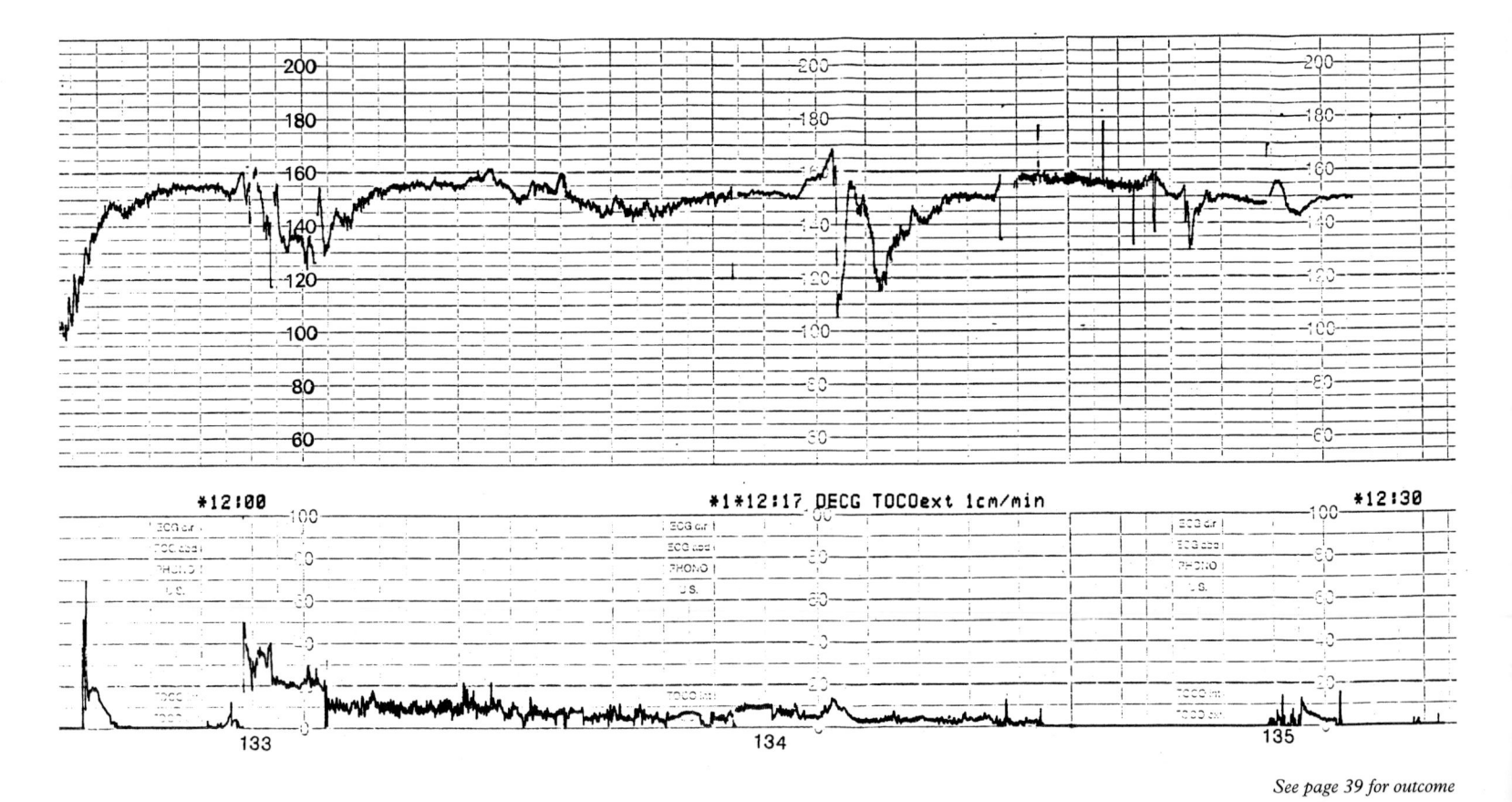

*See page 39 for outcome*

# Outcome

12:35 Emergency caesarean section
ROT position
3.57 kg female
Apgars 9/1 10/5
No cord accident or abruption

No partogram was kept.

**4.1**
Baseline 130–140 bpm; reduced variability, small accelerations.

**4.2**
Baseline 150–160 bpm; trace now more reactive.

**4.3**
There are broad Type 2 decelerations; reasonable variability is maintained within them.

The contraction monitor is showing discoordinate, widely separated contractions.

**4.4**
With persistent decelerations and reduced variability, the decision was taken to proceed to a caesarean section as there was no cervical progress.

Fetal blood sampling would have been very useful in this case. If this had been normal it would then have been reasonable to start oxytocin in this woman. Adequate contractions may have permitted descent and rotation of the fetal head. If the CTG deteriorated and the FBS demonstrated worsening fetal acidosis, it would then have been appropriate to perform a caesarean section.

# Clinical points

### INDICATIONS FOR AN EPIDURAL

— Maternal request
— High risk of instrumental delivery
(e.g. multiple pregnancy, breech
presentation, occipito-posterior
position, previous caesarean section,
fetal distress)
— Pre-eclampsia (platelets and clotting
studies must be normal)
— Stillbirth (abolishes pain and avoids the
mental confusion that may occur with
opiate analgesia; sedatives may still be
given if required)
If use of an epidural is contemplated
antenatally and problems are anticipated, it
is helpful to ask an anaesthetist to see the
mother in order to make preparations for
the labour.

### CONTRAINDICATIONS FOR AN EPIDURAL

— Maternal refusal
— Clotting disorder
— Hypovolaemia
— Sepsis
— Raised intracranial pressure
— Some back and neurological problems

*Cross references:* **Epidurals** *pages 33, 39* **Caesarean section** *page 175* **Fetal blood sampling** *pages 185, 186*

# CASE 5

19-year Moroccan, single, unemployed

Primigravida
No past history

Booked 14 weeks
Anaemic during pregnancy
(haemoglobin between
9–10 g/dl)
Non-smoker

16.5.89 36 + 1 weeks

Admitted with backache
No bleeding
Good growth on scan

Kept in for observation
Daily CTGs reactive with accelerations

# 5.1

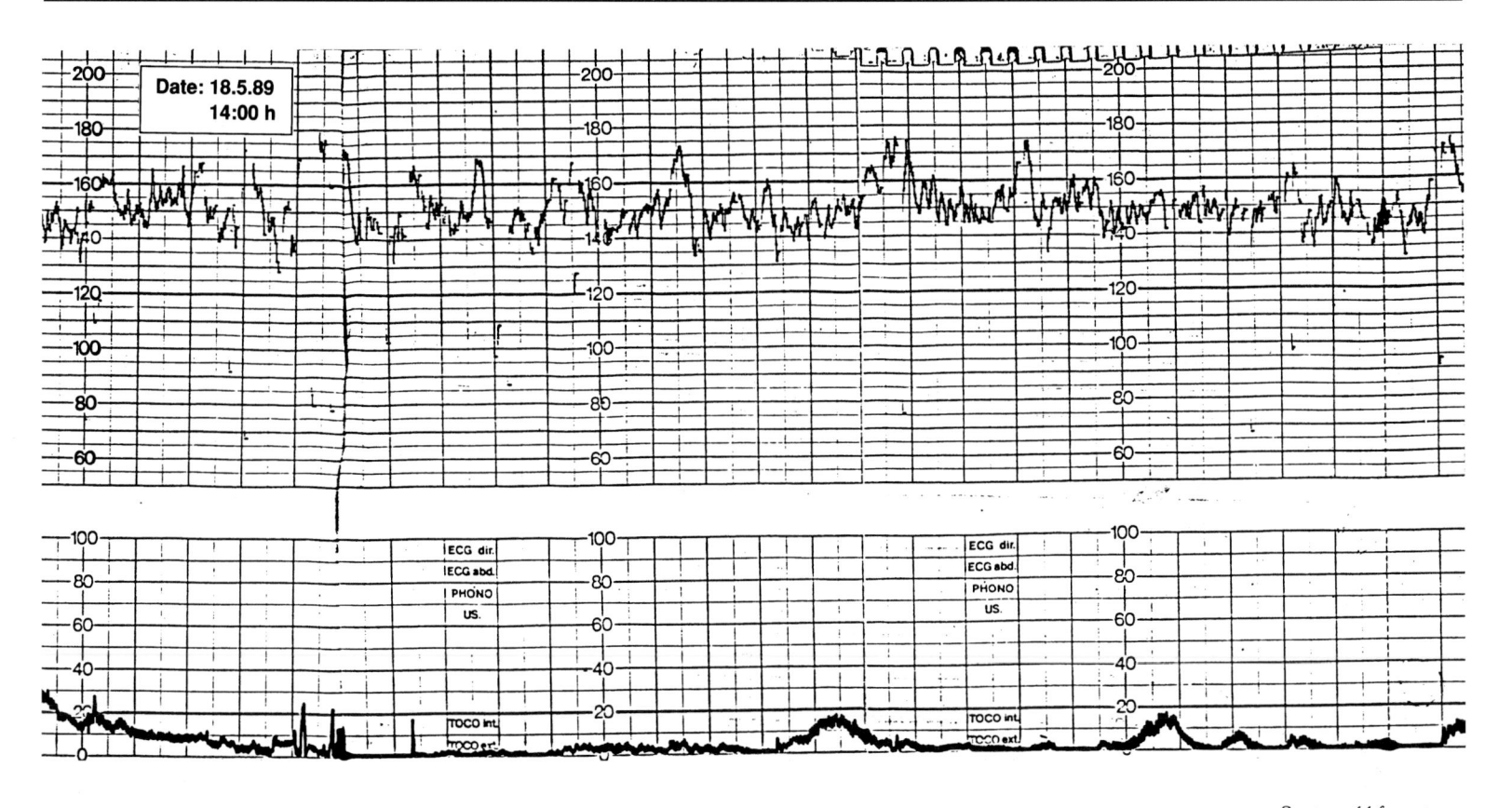

Date: 18.5.89
14:00 h

*See page 44 for outcome*

# 5.2

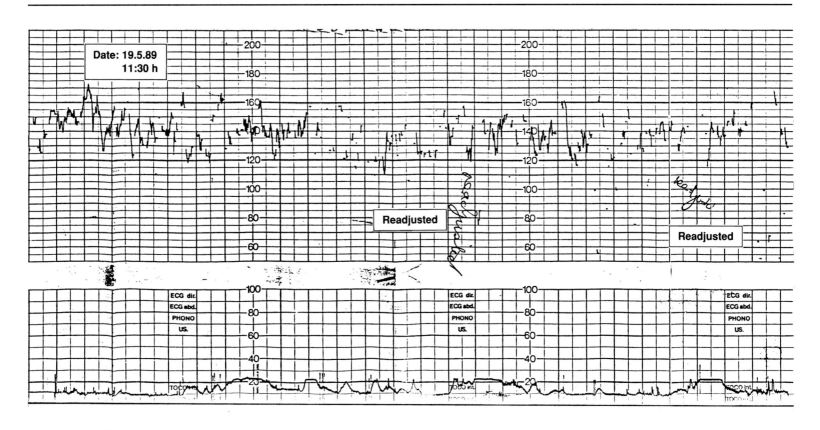

*See page 44 for outcome*

**CASE 5**

# Outcome

20.5.89 Intrauterine death (IUD)
Labour induced with vaginal prostaglandins
2.95 kg female—this is a very good weight for 36 weeks

No partogram was kept.

**5.1**
2 days before the IUD there is good variability with accelerations.

**5.2**
1 day before the IUD the trace is of poor quality. It gives the impression of good reactivity but should really be continued once a good recording is obtained.

Maternal investigations revealed no abnormalities, particularly no evidence of infection or diabetes.

Postmortem showed inhalation of squames suggesting asphyxia. There were no significant abnormalities, and no evidence of placental abruption.

It is difficult to know why this baby died.

# Clinical points

A CTG shows the fetal heart rate at the moment that it is taken and so one must always be cautious about its predictive power. After a normal CTG a sudden deterioration would be unlikely over the next 24 hours, apart from acute insults such as a sudden abruption or cord prolapse.

There are several methods of antepartum monitoring, which will be outlined briefly in this and subsequent cases:

1. Fetal movement monitoring   see opp.
2. Ultrasonography   page 49
3. Biochemical tests   page 59
4. Doppler ultrasound   page 71
5. Cordocentesis   page 86
6. The biophysical profile   page 86
7. The antepartum CTG   pages 49, 81

## FETAL MOVEMENT MONITORING

Keeping a 'kick chart' is a simple way for a mother to assess fetal well-being daily. Although there is a great variation in the individual woman's perception of her baby's movement, over 95 % will be aware of at least ten movements in a 12-hour period. Once the ten movements have been felt (which may be in as little time as half an hour) the mother need count no more until the following day. If fewer than ten movements are felt, or if there is a sudden fall in fetal activity, it is necessary to perform a CTG and possibly check the biophysical profile. A cessation of fetal movement is usually noticed 12–48 hours prior to fetal death. However, not all intrauterine deaths are preceded by a fall in fetal activity.

Fetal movements are greatest at night and early in the morning. The kick chart should therefore be commenced at the same time everyday.

After initial enthusiasm for kick charts, there has recently been some doubt about their overall benefit, largely because of the high incidence of false alarms and also poor compliance in many women with high-risk pregnancies. Most fetal deaths in late pregnancy have an unknown aetiology, and it is thought by some that intervention once there is a reduction in fetal activity, whilst reducing the incidence of antepartum fetal death, has little impact on intrapartum deaths or neonatal morbidity.

Some women find that keeping a kick chart is very stressful, whilst others find it reassuring, and it may enhance bonding. Kick charts should therefore not be given to all women, rather an appropriate form of monitoring should be selected for each individual.

# CASE 6

33-year Asian housewife
Height 1.48 m

G4 P2 +1
1986  NVD 3.3 kg boy
1987  spontaneous miscarriage,
     8 weeks
1988  NVD 3.56 kg girl

No other history

Uncertain dates—EDD by scan
              10.9.89

Booked at 12 weeks

22.9.89 Admitted with decreased fetal movements
      at 41 + 5 weeks

Not in labour
Cephalic presentation
Head 3/5 palpable
Cervix long and closed

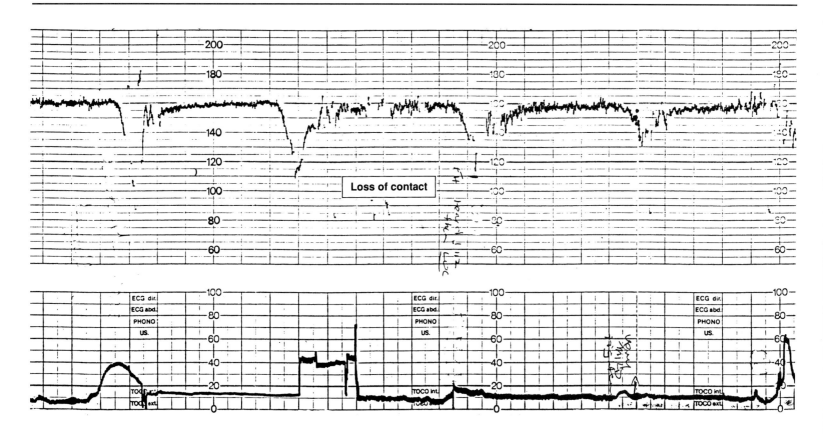

Loss of contact

*See page 48 for outcome*

# Outcome

Shortly after the CTG an emergency caesarean section was performed.
2.87 kg male
No liquor
No cord entanglement or placental abruption
Apgars 2/1 10/5

**6.1**
There was no uterine activity—the CTG picked up very mild tightenings which were neither palpable nor felt by the mother.

There was decreased variability and unprovoked decelerations from a baseline of 160 bpm. The cervix was unfavourable and it was felt that induction of labour would further stress the fetus. The infant was 'post-mature', growth-retarded (note the sizes of her previous babies) and there was no liquor around it. The severe oligohydramnios may have been the cause of the decelerations, as liquor usually prevents undue pressure on the umbilical cord.

This baby's small size was not detected by abdominal palpation in the antenatal clinic. When examining women of small stature from ethnic minorities it is easy to assume that their small baby is normal for them. However, it is as important to exclude placental dysfunction as in any other woman. This is clearly demonstrated in this case by the size of her previous children.

# Clinical points

### The antenatal CTG: 1

In Case 5 we mentioned the limitations of the antenatal CTG. In descriptive terms, the changes from normal that are seen in the compromised fetus are first a reduced overall variability (suboptimal), then the onset of decelerations with some variation still present (decelerative), followed by complete absence of variation with shallower decelerations (terminal) and finally fetal death in utero from asphyxia.

Reduced variability may be due to a fetal rest period—it is unprovoked decelerations that are more sinister. Deeper decelerations are chemoreceptor-mediated vagal bradycardias, which occur in response to acute hypoxia, perhaps superimposed on mild to moderate chronic hypoxia. However, the shallow, smooth decelerations of the 'terminal' trace are predominantly due to non-reflex myocardial depression in the presence of acute on chronic hypoxia.

### Ultrasonography

Ultrasound examination not only detects fetal anomalies but also enables the monitoring of fetal growth, liquor volume and a direct visualization of movement. Fetal movements are seen to become less frequent towards the end of pregnancy, because of the relative reduction in liquor volume compared with the greater space occupied by the fetus itself.

A fall in growth rate can only be determined by serial scans, which should be at least 2 weeks apart in order to demonstrate a significant change. If facilities permit, a routine scan at 32–34 weeks' gestation enables early detection of the small-for-dates fetus, at a time when more intensive monitoring can be instituted. This may allow appropriate intervention and a reduction in perinatal morbidity.

A reduction in liquor volume (oligohydramnios) is seen in association with fetal anomalies (e.g. renal agenesis, posterior urethral valves), premature rupture of the membranes (a diagnosis not always suggested by the history) and intrauterine growth retardation (in which it is a poor prognostic sign).

An ultrasound scan early in the third trimester of this woman's pregnancy probably would have alerted us to a fetus that was small for gestational age and would have prompted serial ultrasound tracking of fetal growth. A decision to induce labour may have been reached before the oligohydramnios had developed, thus avoiding an operative delivery in this multiparous woman.

*Cross references:* **Antenatal monitoring** *pages 45, 59, 71, 81, 86*

# CASE 7

35-year Jamaican, single,
unemployed

G3 P0 +2 (TOPs)
No other history

EDD 9.6.90

Booked 12 weeks

9.6.90   40 weeks

05:15   Admitted in labour with spontaneous
        rupture of membranes
        Cephalic presentation
        Left occipito-transverse (LOT) position
        Head 2/5 palpable abdominally
        Cervix 5 cm dilated
        Head LOT
        Clear liquor
        Pethidine given

09:25   7 cm

10:20   Pethidine
        7 cm
        Oxytocin commenced

11:45   Fully dilated

# 7.1

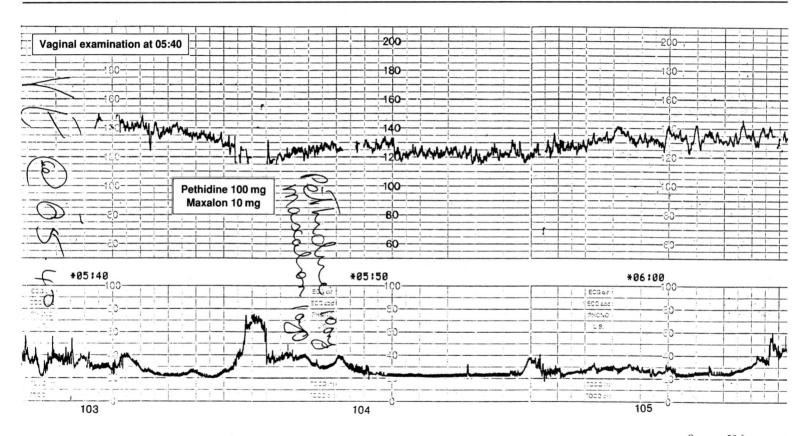

Vaginal examination at 05:40

Pethidine 100 mg
Maxalon 10 mg

*05:40   *05:50   *06:00

103   104   105

*See page 58 for outcome*

# 7.2

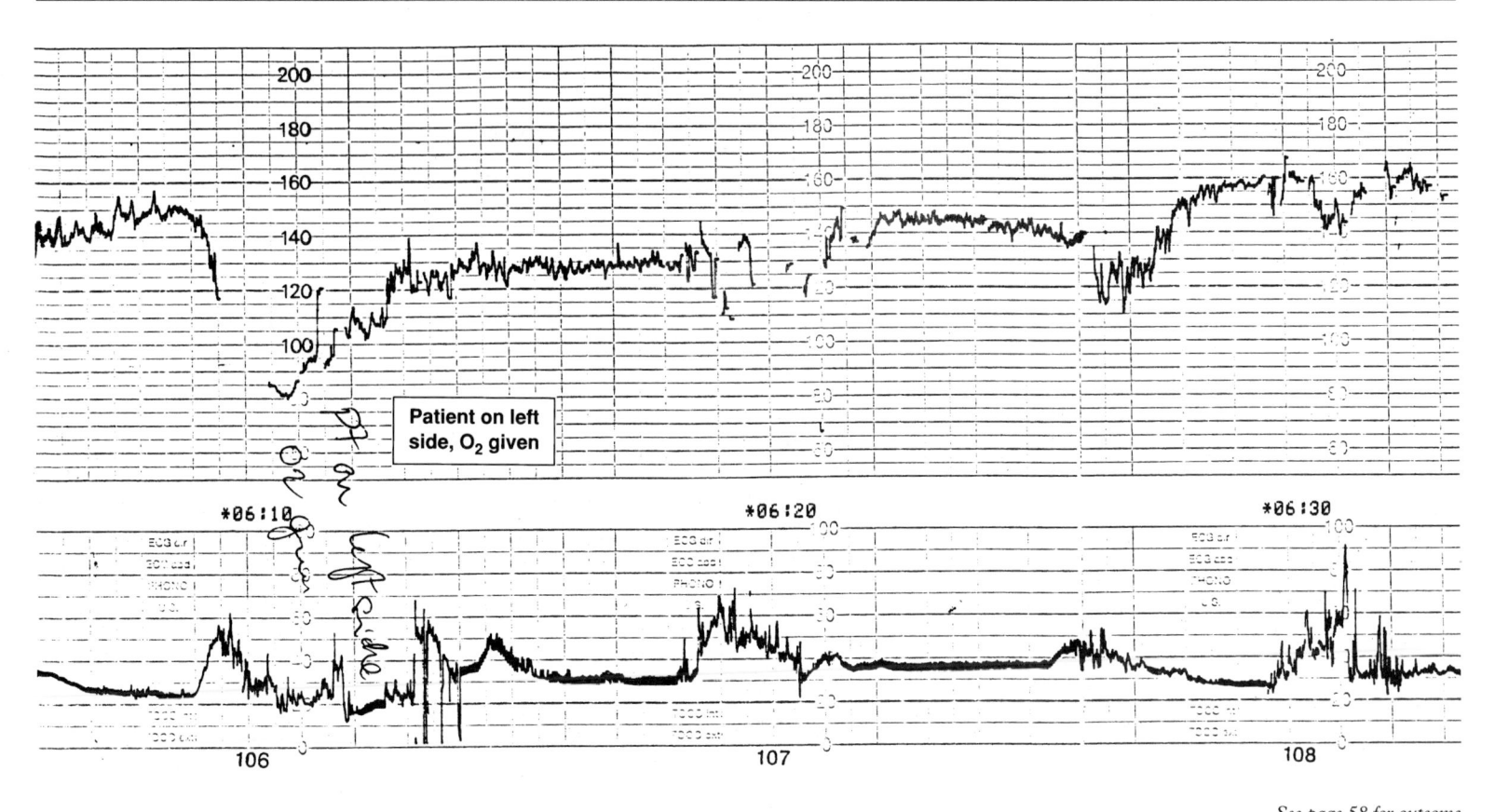

Patient on left side, O₂ given

*See page 58 for outcome*

# 7.3

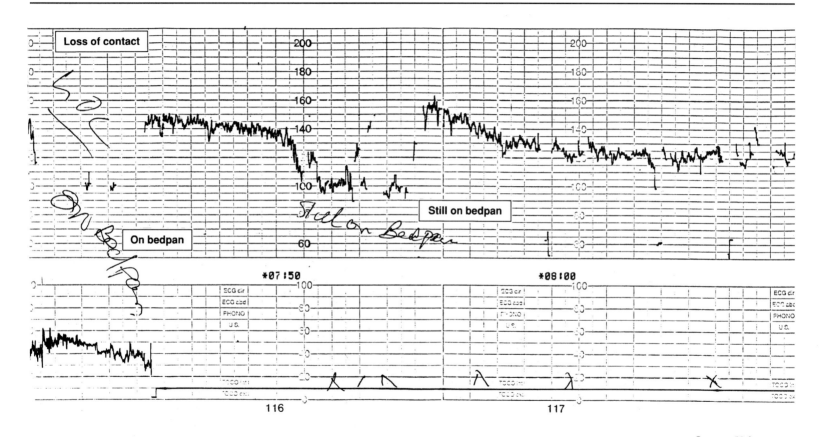

Loss of contact

On bedpan

Still on bedpan

*07:50  *08:00

116  117

*See page 58 for outcome*

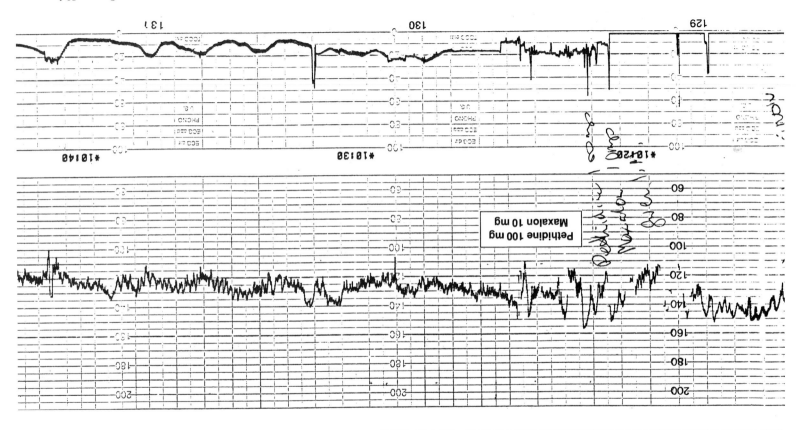

Pethidine 100 mg
Maxalon 10 mg

7.4

# 7.5

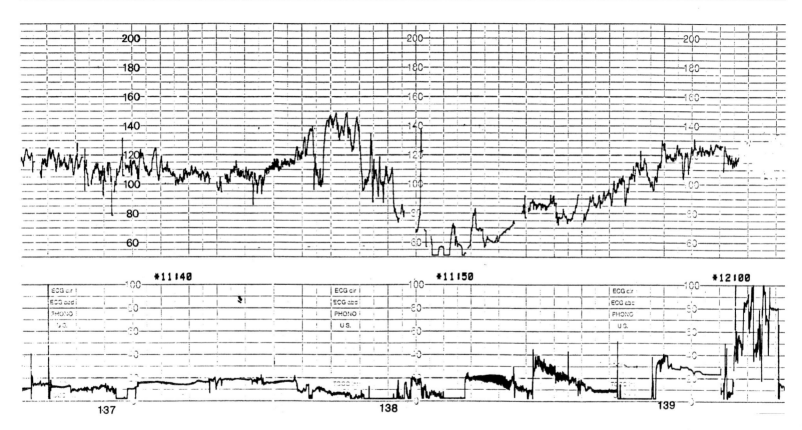

*See page 58 for outcome*

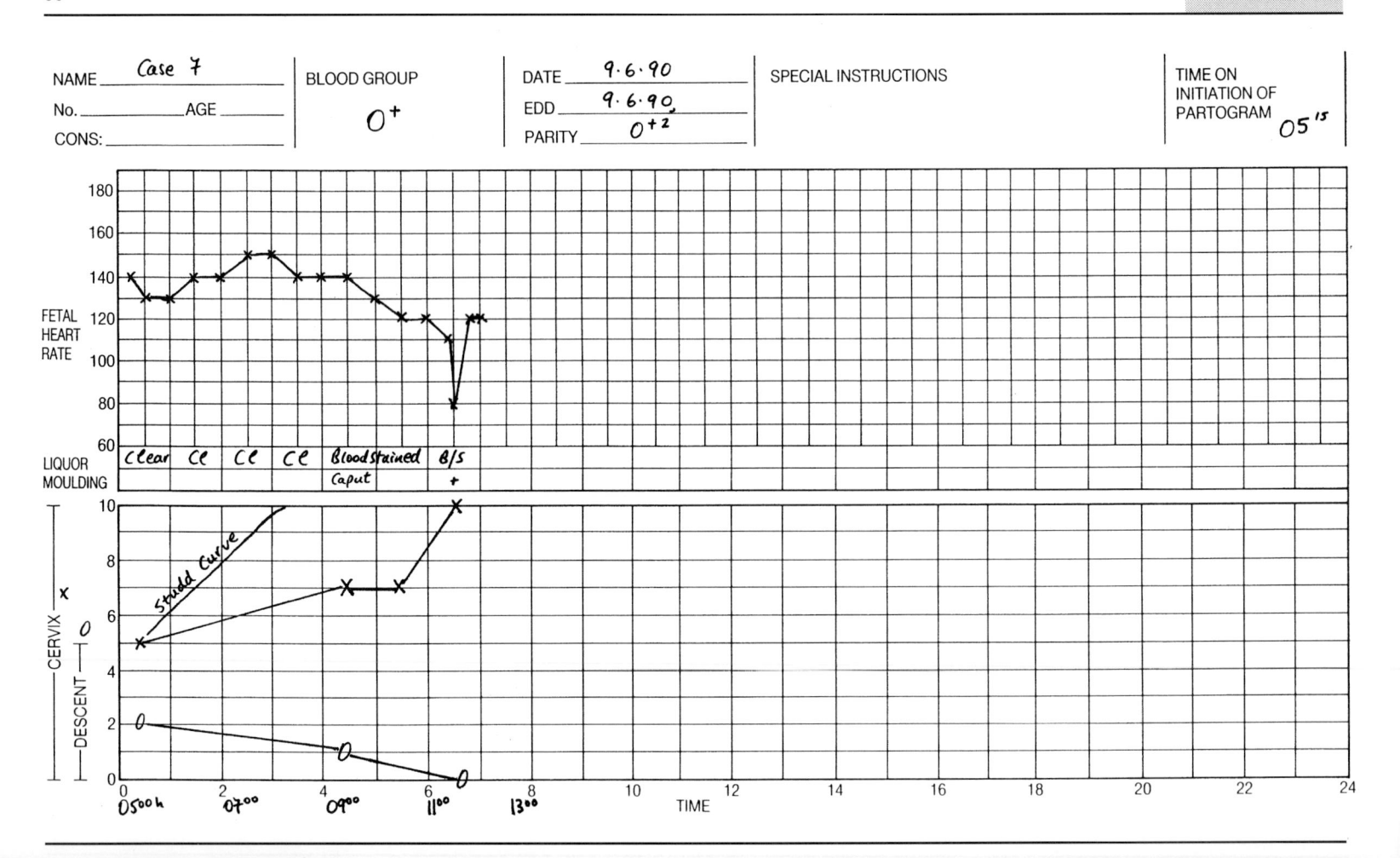

NAME __Case 7__

No. _____ AGE _____

CONS: _____

BLOOD GROUP

$O^+$

DATE __9.6.90__

EDD __9.6.90__

PARITY __$0^{+2}$__

SPECIAL INSTRUCTIONS

TIME ON INITIATION OF PARTOGRAM __$05^{15}$__

FETAL HEART RATE

180
160
140
120
100
80
60

LIQUOR MOULDING

Clear | Cℓ | Cℓ | Cℓ | Blood Stained / Caput | B/S / +

CERVIX

DESCENT

Studd Curve

10
8
6
4
2
0

0 | 2 | 4 | 6 | 8 | 10 | 12 | 14 | 16 | 18 | 20 | 22 | 24

$05^{00}$ h | $07^{00}$ | $09^{00}$ | $11^{00}$ | $13^{00}$

TIME

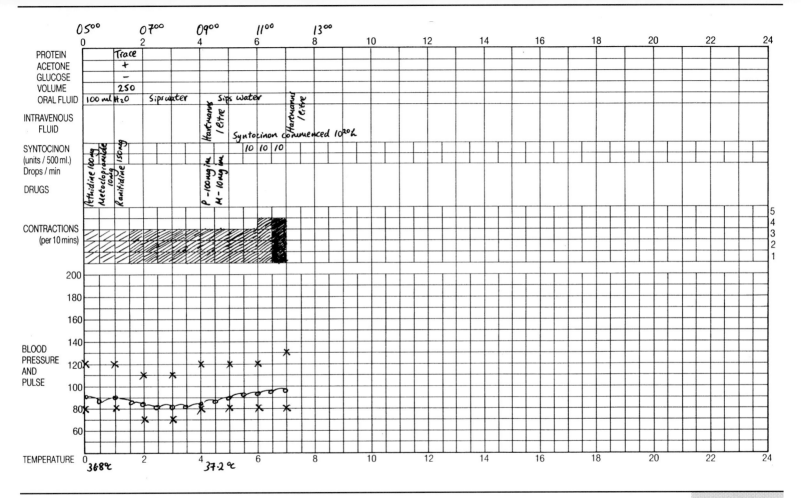

# Outcome

12:00    Neville-Barnes forceps delivery
Left occipito-anterior, caput ++
3.4 kg female
Shoulder dystocia at delivery
Apgars 4/1 9/5 10/10
Right Erb's palsy (this later
recovered completely)

**7.1**
Baseline 120–130 bpm, reactive.

**7.2**
The baseline is rising after prolonged
Type 2 decelerations.

**7.3**
The baseline has settled at 130–140 bpm;
there is a further bradycardic episode. The
Xs represent uterine contractions when the
belt is either off or not working.

**7.4**
The trace is more reactive now with
accelerations. Oxytocin is commenced for
slow progress.

**7.5**
Baseline has fallen to 110 bpm; there is
then a prolonged bradycardia. At full
dilatation a forceps delivery was performed.
There were no predictors for the shoulder
dystocia which then occurred.

# Clinical points

## SHOULDER DYSTOCIA

Shoulder dystocia is classically said to occur in women who are having a prolonged labour and have risk factors for a large baby, such as gestational diabetes or a previous large baby. However, as in this case, 50 % of babies who have this serious complication weigh less than 4 kg. Unfortunately there are no reliable antenatal predictors.

The diagnosis becomes apparent when the head delivers but the shoulders become stuck. It is vital first to ensure that the shoulders have rotated into the antero-posterior plane of the pelvic outlet. A large episiotomy is required, the mother's legs should be abducted (by taking them out of the lithotomy poles and flexing them against the abdomen the anterior shoulder may be released) and an assistant should also press suprapubically to try and disempact the anterior shoulder. If the anterior shoulder cannot then be delivered it should be possible to deliver the posterior shoulder and arm and the anterior shoulder and trunk will then follow.

Care should be taken to avoid a brachial plexus injury or a fractured clavicle, although if either should occur, recovery is often complete. Indeed, sometimes a clavicle is deliberately broken to expedite delivery. If the above measures fail to deliver the baby it is possible to procede to a symphysiotomy, or, in extreme circumstances, to push the head back into the vagina and rapidly perform a caesarean section.

## ANTENATAL MONITORING: 3

### Biochemical tests
It used to be popular to measure biochemical parameters of placental function, which were thought to provide information about the preceding weeks rather than only at the time of the test. Substances measured included oestriol, human placental lactogen, human chorionic gonadotrophin and alpha fetoprotein. None of these is able to provide a reliable sensitivity for fetal compromise. The measurement of various placental proteins is still being researched and may prove to be useful in the future.

Cross references:   **Antenatal monitoring**  pages 45, 49, 71, 81, 86

CASE 7

# CASE 8

20-year Indian housewife

Primigravida
No past history

LMP 10.10.89–EDD 17.7.90

Booked 16 weeks
Shared care
Uneventful pregnancy until
36 weeks

20.6.90 36 weeks
Admitted with raised blood pressure
3+ proteinuria, oedema
Decreased fetal growth (fetal abdominal
circumference on 5th centile)
Cephalic presentation

24.6.90 Blood pressure (BP) had been stable
/90–/100 diastolic
Now increase in BP to 170/130 and vomiting

23:30 Hydralazine bolus and infusion
Chlormethiazole infusion
Prostaglandin $E_2$ gel (1 mg) inserted

05:30 BP stable
Further prostaglandin gel (2 mg)

Throughout the morning maternal condition was
stable although labour did not start.

# 8.1

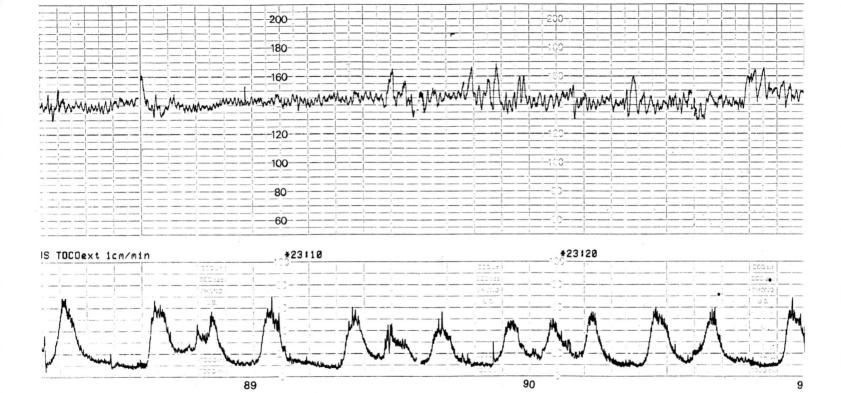

IS TOCOext 1cm/min        *23110             *23120

89                  90            9

*See page 70 for outcome*

# 8.2

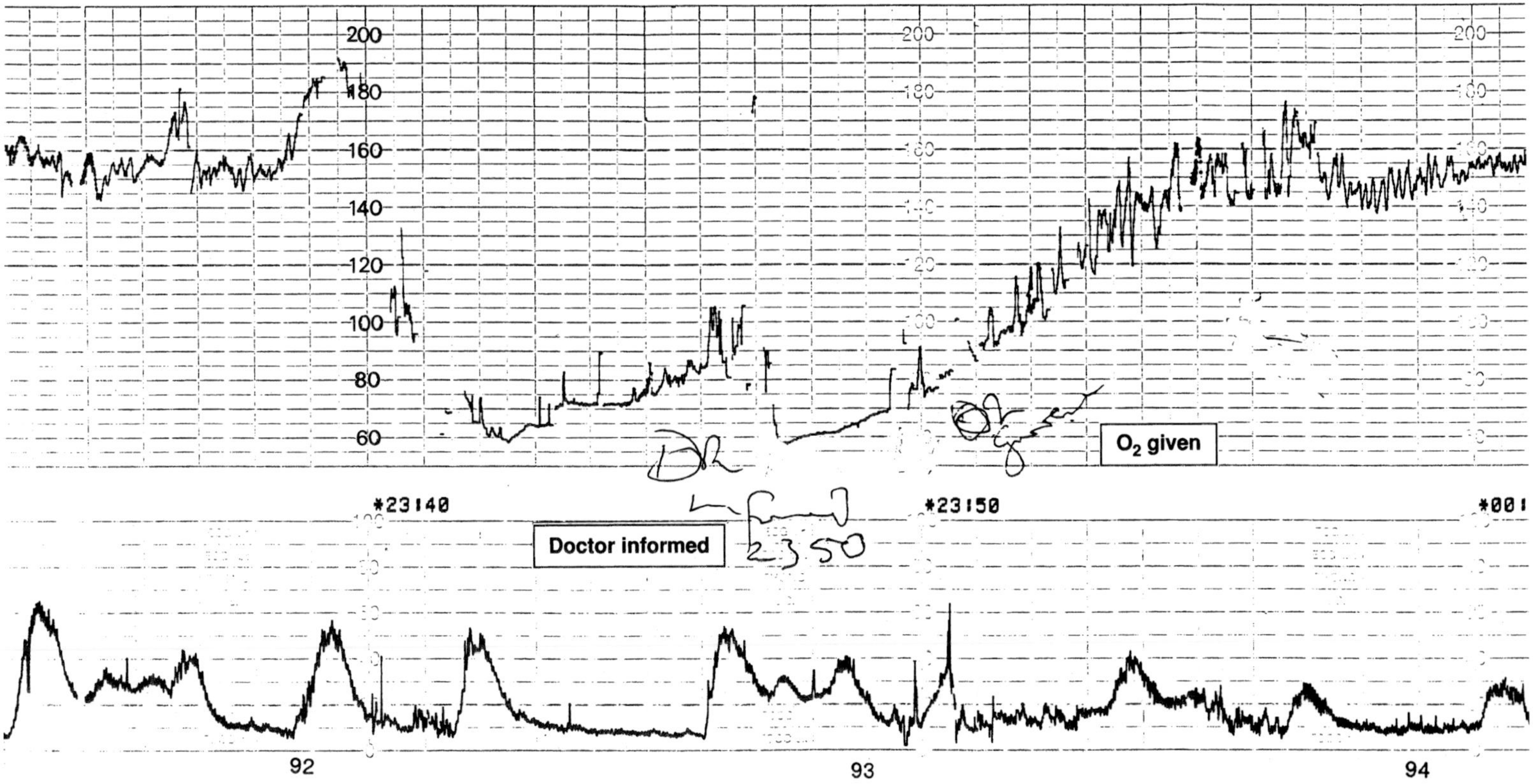
200
180
160
140
120
100
80
60
*23140
*23150
*001
Doctor informed
O$_2$ given
92
93
94

*See page 70 for outcome*

# 8.3

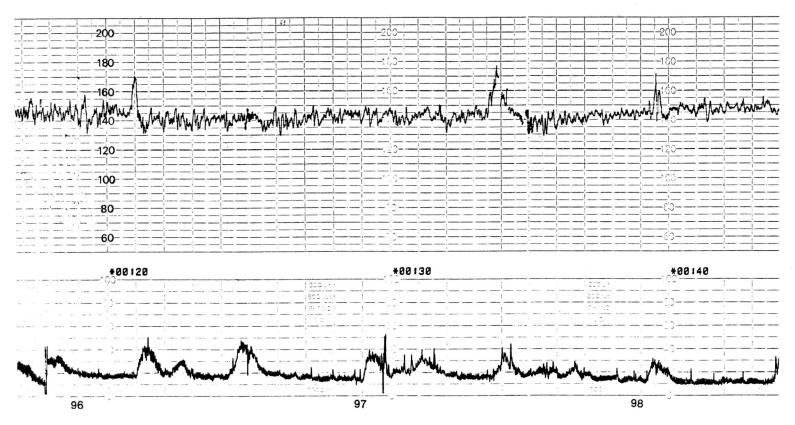

*See page 70 for outcome*

CASE 8

# 8.4

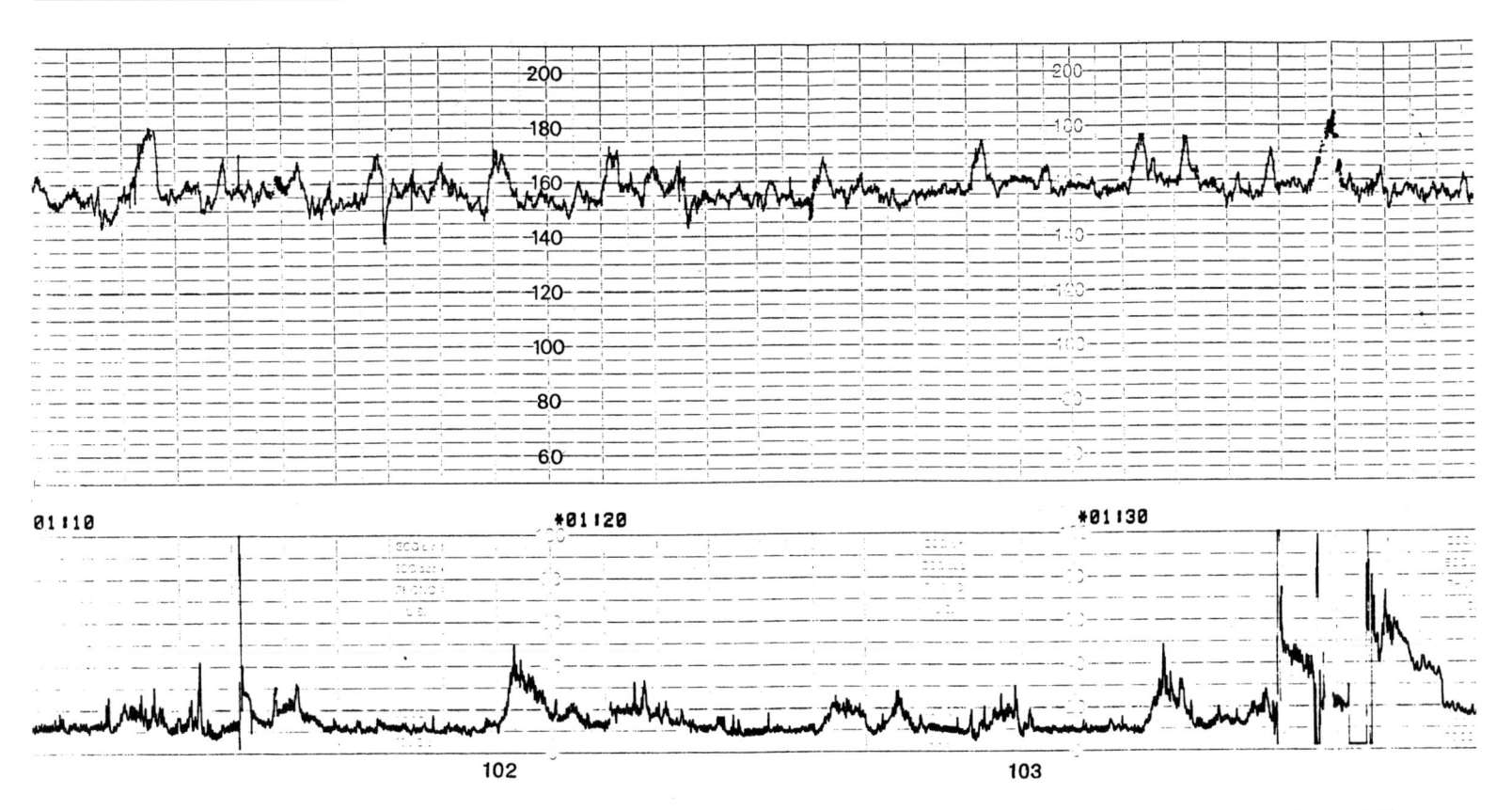

*See page 70 for outcome*

# 8.5

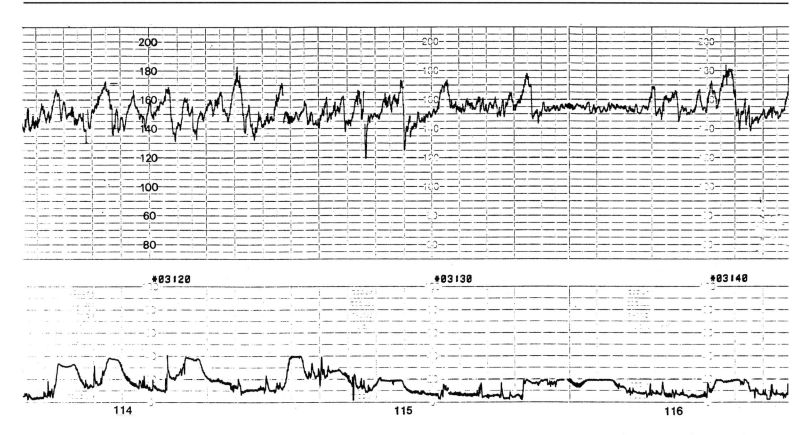

*See page 70 for outcome*

# 8.6

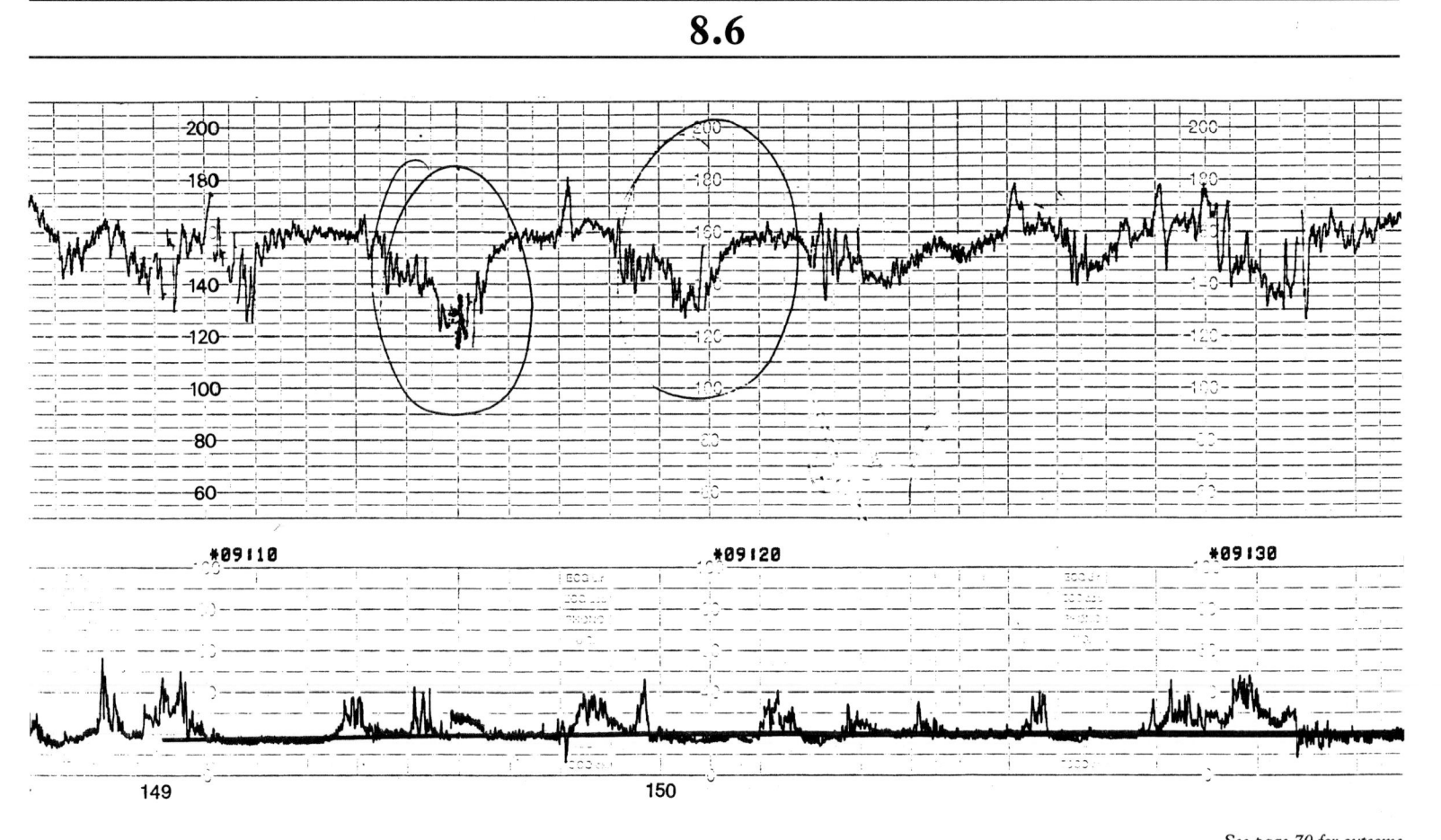

*See page 70 for outcome*

# 8.7

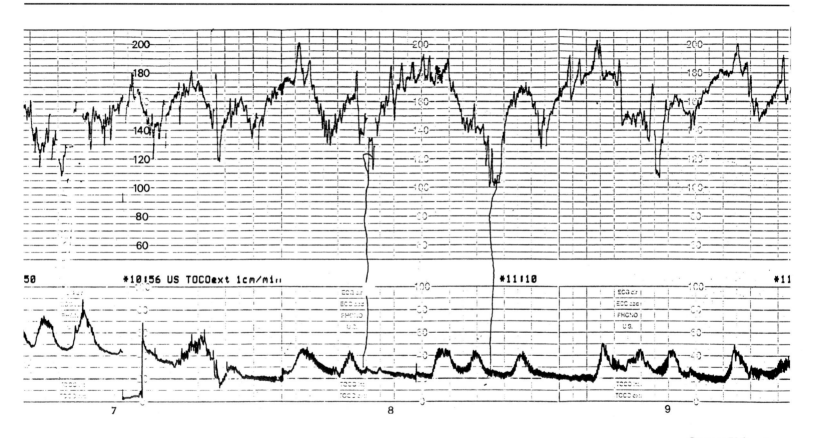

*See page 70 for outcome*

# 8.8

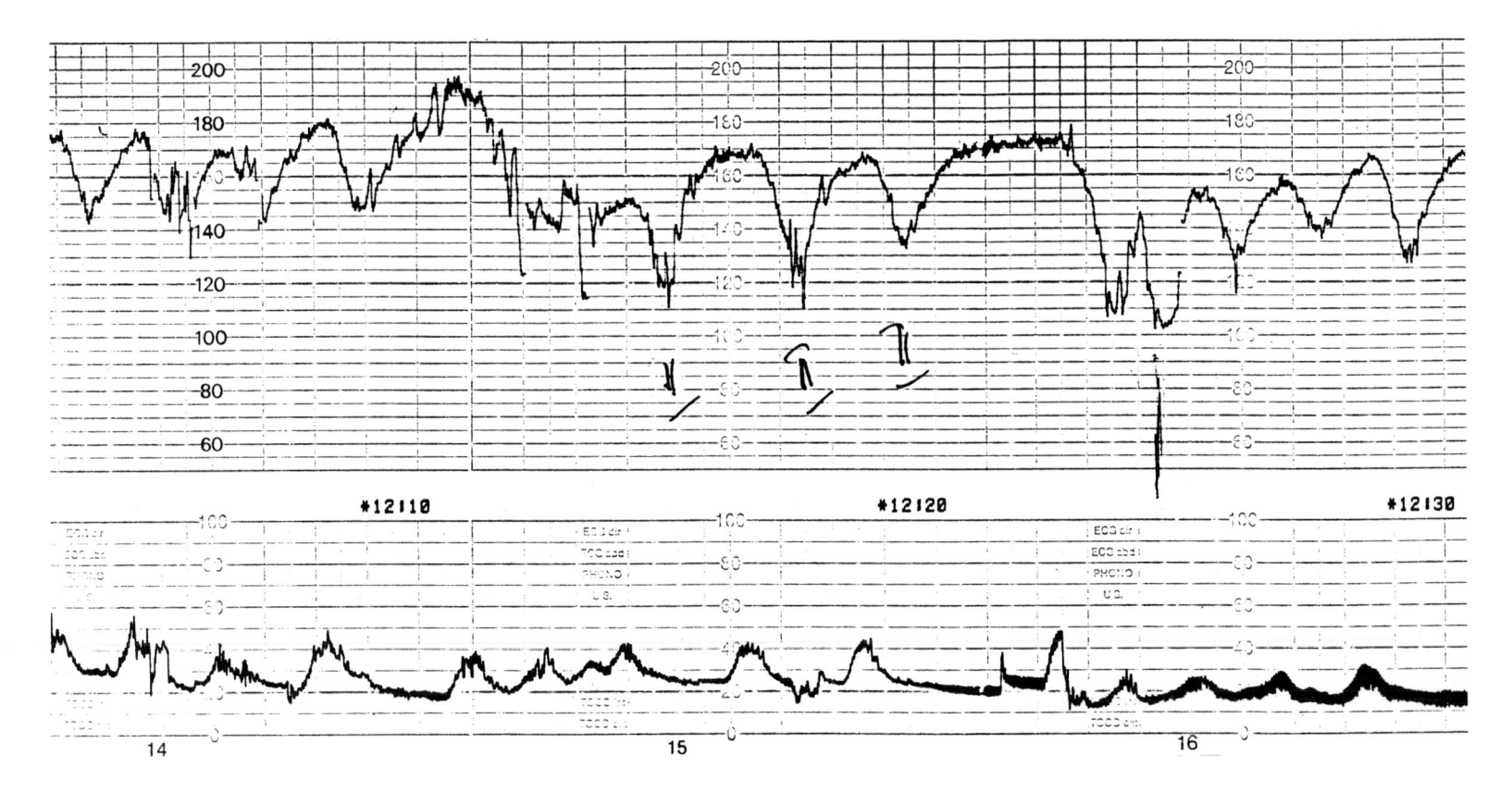

*See page 70 for outcome*

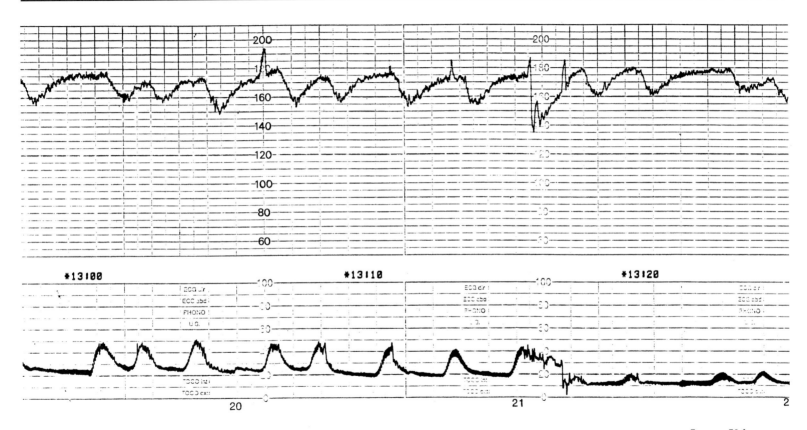

*See page 70 for outcome*

# Outcome

15:30    Emergency caesarean section
under epidural
Clear liquor, left occipito-
transverse position
2.7 kg male (not a bad size for
36 weeks)
Apgars 9/1 10/5

This was a worrying case of severe
proteinuric pre-eclampsia at 36 weeks'
gestation. The decision was taken to try
and induce labour. Sometimes this is
surprisingly rapid in pre-eclamptics.

**8.1**
Prior to prostaglandin: baseline 140 bpm,
good variability and accelerations. Uterine
activity suggests that induction may be
easy, yet these contractions were not felt by
the mother.

**8.2**
This prolonged deceleration would have
been worrying had there not been a reactive
trace before and after. There is also some
variability within the deceleration itself. It
was thought to be due to either the
unpredictable absorption of a bolus of
prostaglandin gel, causing a hypertonic
contraction, or secondary to the fall in blood
pressure induced by an accidental bolus of
hydralazine, although a continuous
hydralazine infusion may cause a
tachycardia.

**8.3**
Following the deceleration there is good
variability and accelerations and so it was
considered safe to continue.

**8.4**
This is a healthy reactive trace. The
baseline is now 150–160 bpm—possibly a
hydralazine effect causing both maternal
and fetal tachycardia.

**8.5**
Still good variability and accelerations.

**8.6**
These decelerations are Type 2; there is
still minimal uterine activity.

**8.7**
The baseline has risen further to
170–180 bpm and the Type 2 decelerations
persist; variability remains good but the
fetus is probably distressed.

**8.8 & 8.9**
There is now reduced variability with
continued late decelerations. The induction
had failed, but caesarean delivery was
delayed because of parental opposition.

# Clinical points

## HYPERTONIC CONTRACTIONS

These may occur after a bolus, or too high a dose of prostaglandins or oxytocin, and also when there is CPD, particularly in multiparous women. If the contraction persists and the fetal heart rate drops, one should stop the oxytocin infusion and administer oxygen. Sometimes it is necessary to give an intravenous tocolytic, such as salbutamol, to relax the uterus. If there is continuing fetal distress, the baby should be delivered.

## ANTENATAL MONITORING: 4

Induction of labour was necessary in this patient because of a deteriorating maternal condition. Had this not been the case, it would have been possible to look for other criteria of fetal compromise to decide upon the urgency for delivery. The ultrasound scan demonstrated a reduced abdominal circumference and normal liquor volume, yet this was a single measurement and only serial scans can distinguish between a baby that is growth retarded because of placental dysfunction and a 'normally small' baby.

### Doppler ultrasound

This employs the same principal as the external heart rate transducer, but in addition examines the velocity of blood flow by computing the difference between the transmitted ultrasound wave and its reflected signal. In this way the characteristics of the blood flow in the uteroplacental and fetal circulations can be assessed. The vessels that are usually examined are the uterine and umbilical arteries, although the fetal aorta and carotid arteries may also be studied.

Flow should be forwards in both systole and diastole. If there is resistance to flow, as seen in intrauterine growth retardation and/or pre-eclampsia, the diastolic wave form is first impeded at the end of diastole, it then disappears and in severe cases becomes reversed. Various mathematical ratios have been evolved to express the relationship between systolic and diastolic flow, but clinical assessment is based upon the presence or absence of end-diastolic flow or its reversal. There has been a plethora of research in this field in recent years, yet the role of Doppler studies within the armamentarium of antenatal assessment has yet to be fully defined.

Cross references:   **Antenatal monitoring**  *pages 45, 49, 59, 81, 86*

# CASE 9

16-year

Primigravida

EDD 3.7.90
Booked 18 weeks

Uneventful pregnancy

4.7.90   40+ weeks

14:30   Admitted in labour
        Cephalic presentation
        Left occipito-anterior position
        Head 2/5 palpable
        Cervix 2 cm dilated
        Membranes intact

16:00   2 cm

19:00   4 cm
        Amniotomy, clear liquor

21:00   5 cm
        Good contractions

22:00   7–8 cm

24:00   9 cm

24:30   Fully dilated

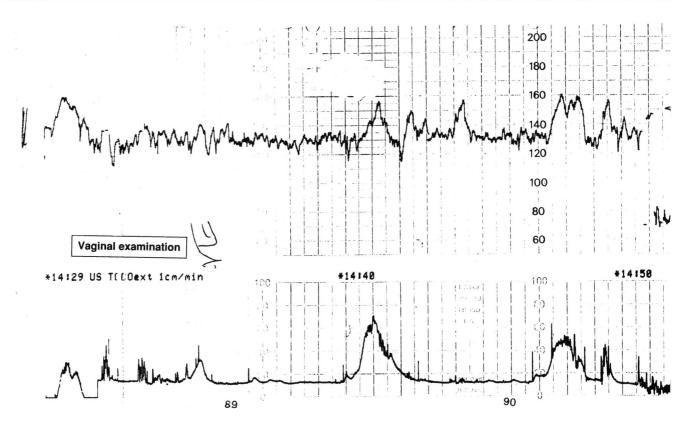

Vaginal examination

*14:29 US T(CO)ext 1cm/min

*See page 80 for outcome*

# 9.2

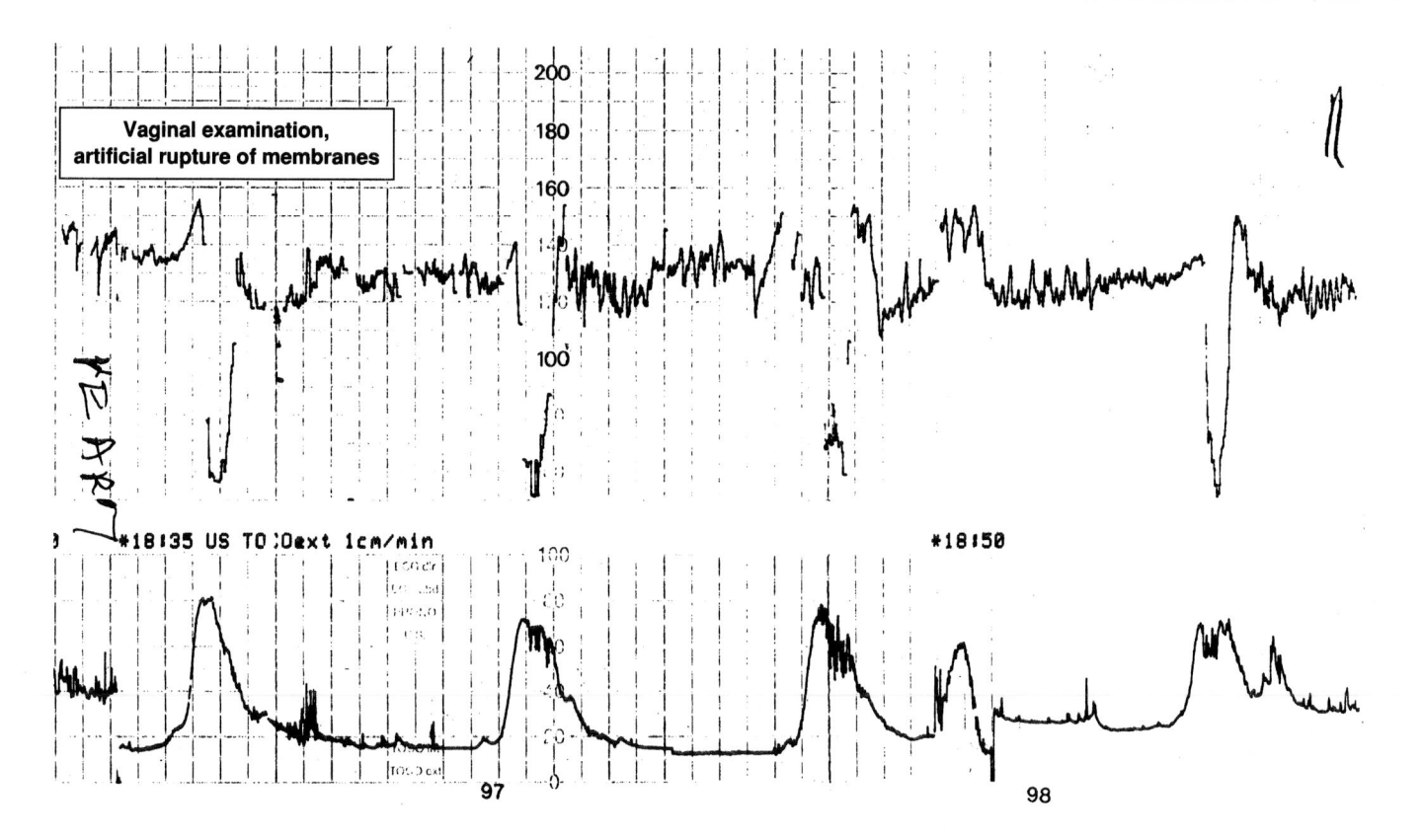

Vaginal examination, artificial rupture of membranes

*See page 80 for outcome*

# 9.3

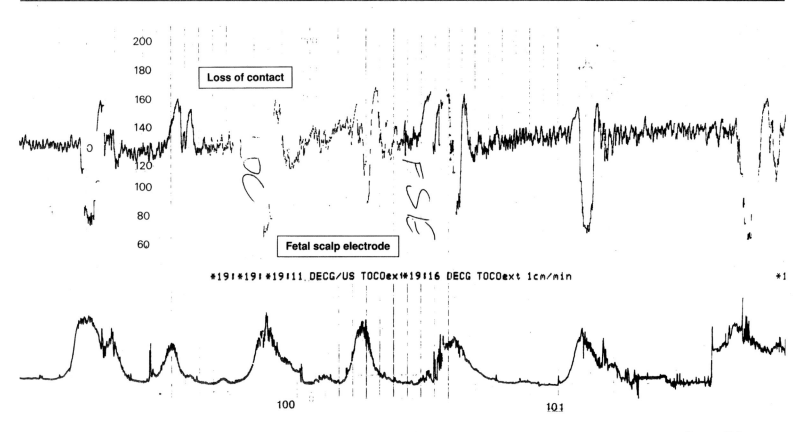

Loss of contact

Fetal scalp electrode

*19ı*19ı*19ı11 DECG/US TOCOext*19ı16 DECG TOCOext 1cm/min    *1

*See page 80 for outcome*

# 9.4

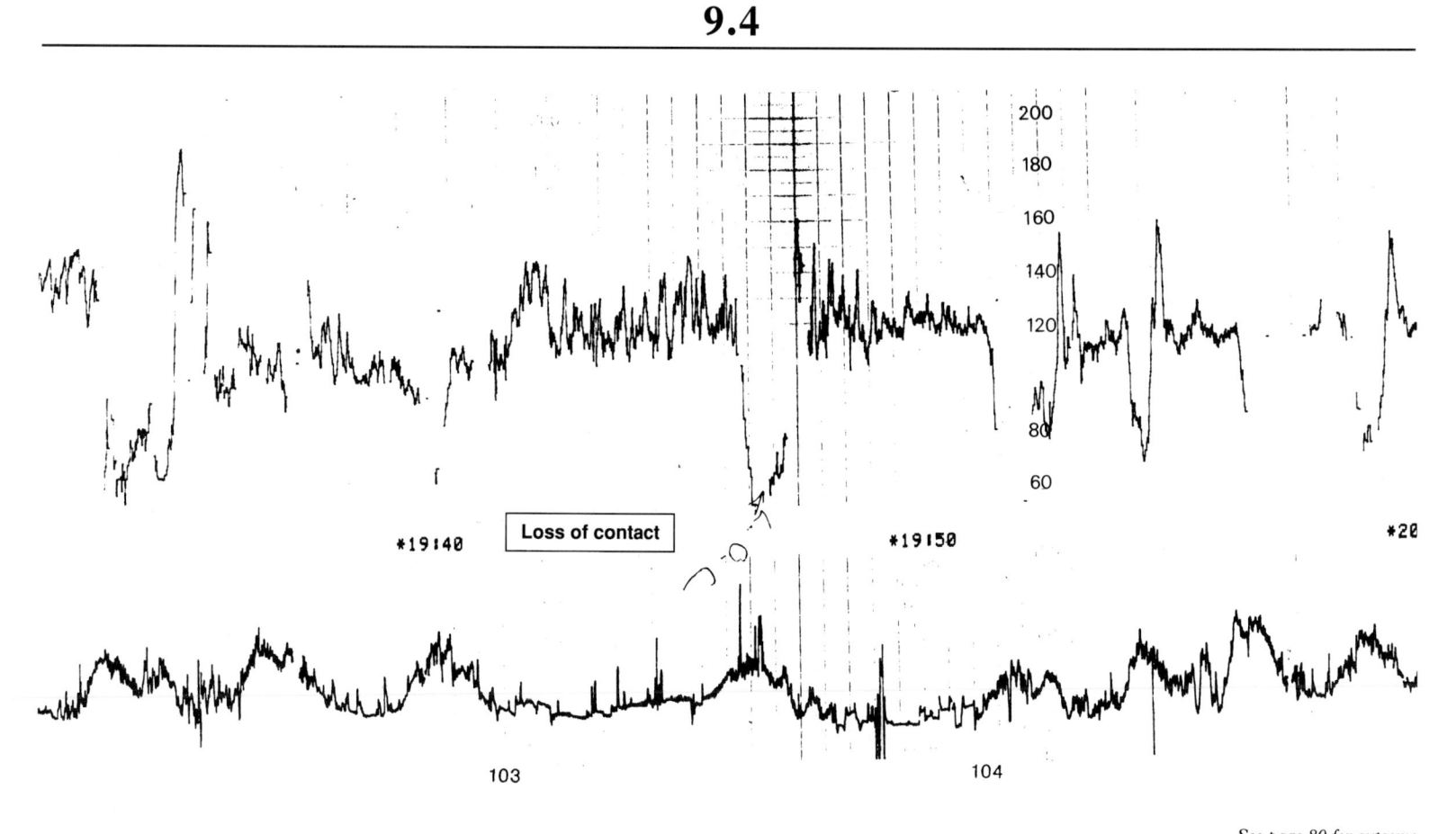

Loss of contact

*19:40    *19:50    *20

103    104

*See page 80 for outcome*

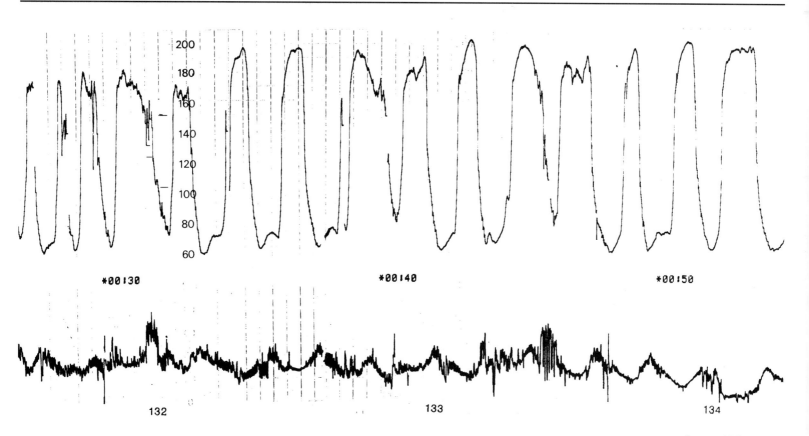

*00130          *00140          *00150

132          133          134

*See page 80 for outcome*

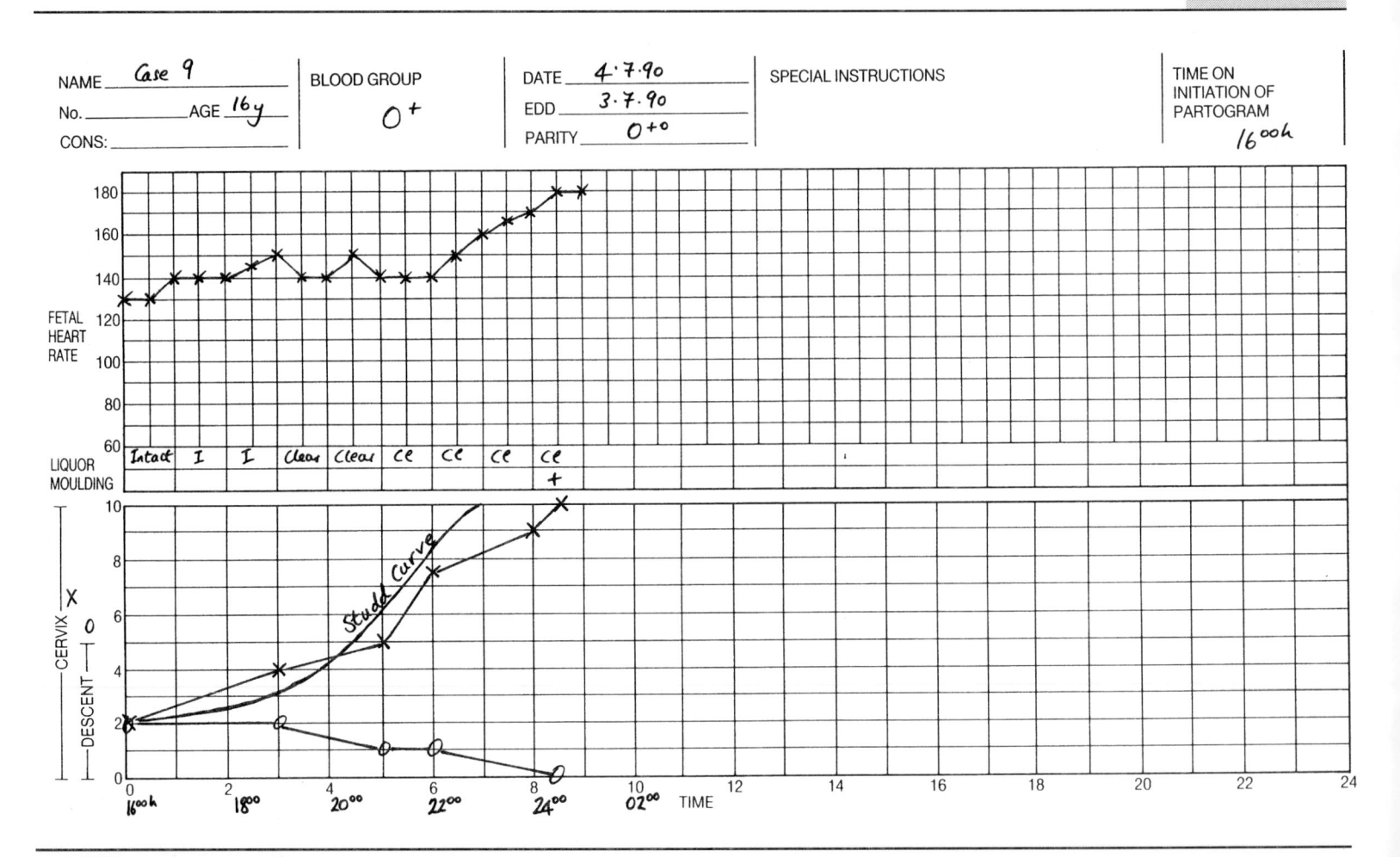

NAME _Case 9_

No. _____ AGE _16y_

CONS: _____

BLOOD GROUP

_O +_

DATE _4.7.90_

EDD _3.7.90_

PARITY _0 +0_

SPECIAL INSTRUCTIONS

TIME ON
INITIATION OF
PARTOGRAM

_16°°h_

FETAL
HEART
RATE

180
160
140
120
100
80
60

LIQUOR
MOULDING

| Intact | I | I | Clear | Clear | Ce | Ce | Ce | Ce |
|        |   |   |       |       |    |    |    | +  |

CERVIX — X
DESCENT — O

10
8
6
4
2
0

Stude Curve

TIME

0   16°°h   2   18°°   4   20°°   6   22°°   8   24°°   10   02°°   12   14   16   18   20   22   24

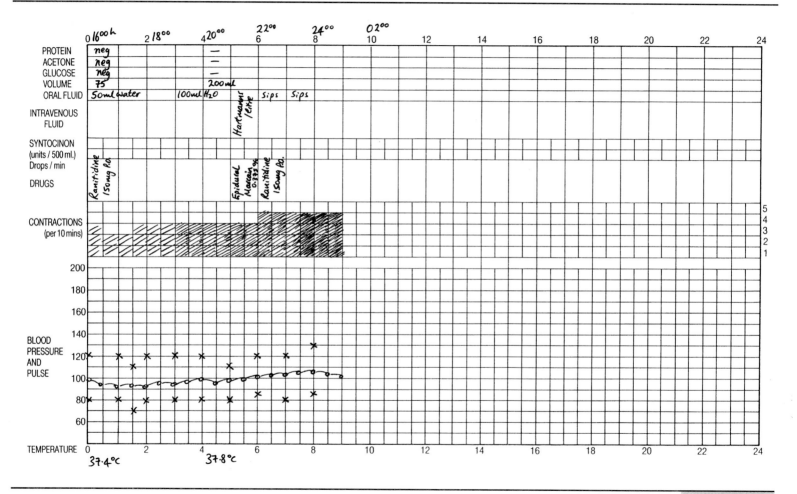

# Outcome

01:00    Spontaneous delivery
2.5 kg female
Apgars 6/1 8/5 10/10
Cord once around neck,
meconium behind head

**9.1**
Reactive trace, baseline 130 bpm.

**9.2**
Good variability; deep Type 1
decelerations with accelerations after; this
is probably due to cord compression.

**9.3 & 9.4**
Accelerations either side of decelerations
are a good sign, but the decelerations
continue to be deep and there are some
Type 2s. This continued for several hours
and labour progressed slowly.

**9.5**
This is a very ominous trace; the mother
was in the second stage, but there is a
dramatic decompensation in heart rate and
no variability.

The baby delivered spontaneously, but was
distressed and there was meconium behind
the head that was not discovered until
birth. In retrospect, this baby should have
been delivered earlier, particularly as fetal
blood sampling was not available to refute
the CTG appearances of hypoxia.

# Clinical points

## The Antenatal CTG: 2

In the discussion after Case 6 we outlined the progressive deterioration that may be seen on the antenatal CTG prior to fetal death (page 49). Although the CTG simply represents the fetal heart rate during the time that it is being recorded, a healthy trace indicates that the fetus is at low risk over the next 24–48 hours. Ways of providing an extrapolated prognosis of fetal well-being include scoring the CTG and stressing the fetus during the CTG. A popular scoring system is the modified Fischer score, in which a score of 8–10 is normal, 5–7 suspicious and less than 5 abnormal.

Normal scores are fairly reliable predictors of good outcome. An abnormal score indicates the need for more detailed evaluation. Of the different parameters it is the presence of decelerations that is most

|  | Score 2 | 1 | 0 |
|---|---|---|---|
| Baseline rate (bpm) | 120–160 | 100–120 160–180 | <100, >180 |
| Amplitude of variability (bpm) | 10–25 | 5–10 25 | <5 sinusoidal |
| Oscillation frequency (cycles/minute) | >4 | 2–4 | <2 sinusoidal |
| Accelerations with fetal movements or stimulation | + | atypical shape | – |
| Decelerations with Braxton Hicks uterine contractions | – or type 1 | <25% late or mild/mod. variable | >25% late or severe variable |

worrying whilst the baseline rate contributes least to the prognosis. Unfortunately there are still a significant number of false positive results, and the system does not take account of rest-activity cycling behaviour (pages 2–3). Dogmatic adherence to the score may thus lead to unnecessary intervention.

Additional tests have been devised which are designed to stress the fetus in order to determine how well it will stand up to the rigours of labour. Such stress tests involve either an oxytocin infusion to induce uterine contractions, or nipple stimulation to induce natural oxytocin production. These procedures are potentially dangerous because of the difficulty in controlling the oxytocin load and the consequent risk of causing hypertonic contractions or the start of labour. Apart from this, the contraction stress test has not become popular, largely because of its poor overall diagnostic ability and practical difficulties. Acoustic stimulation is another provocative test which is free from the above dangers, and some studies have suggested that an accelerative fetal heart rate response, both before and during labour, augurs well for neonatal health.

*Cross references:* **Meconium** *pages 33, 118* **Antenatal monitoring** *pages 45, 49, 59, 71, 86* **Fetal blood sampling** *pages 185, 186*

# CASE 10

37-year single, social worker

Primigravida
No past history
Non-smoker

Uncertain dates—by scan EDD
12.7.89

Booked at 18 weeks—too late
for amniocentesis

17.5.89 32 weeks, decreased fetal movements
26-week size, scan: growth under 5th centile

18.5.89 Worrying CTG
Referred to Queen Charlotte's Maternity Hospital
Biophysical profile score 8/10
Doppler studies—absent umbilical artery
end-diastolic flow
Scan suggested an abnormal heart
Fetal blood sampling
— pH 7.27 (normal 7.35)
— base excess: -8.6 mmol/l (normal up to -10)
— karyotype normal
Cardiac scan at Guy's Hospital—
mild cardiomegaly

20.5.89 Plan to stay in for daily monitoring

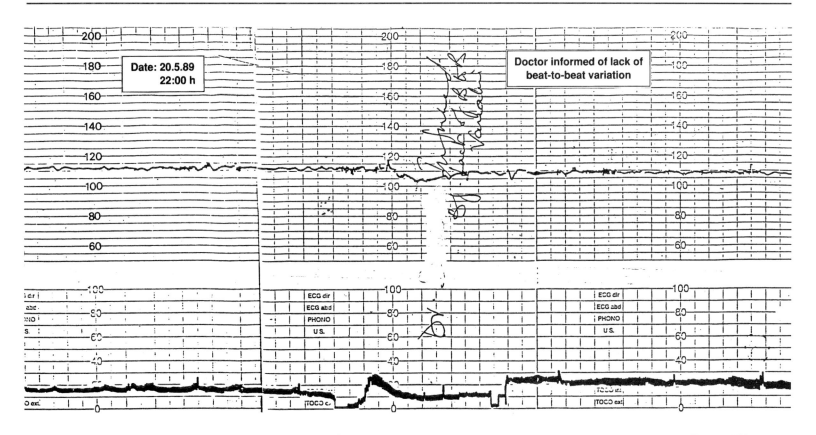

Date: 20.5.89
22:00 h

Doctor informed of lack of
beat-to-beat variation

*See page 85 for outcome*

## 10.2

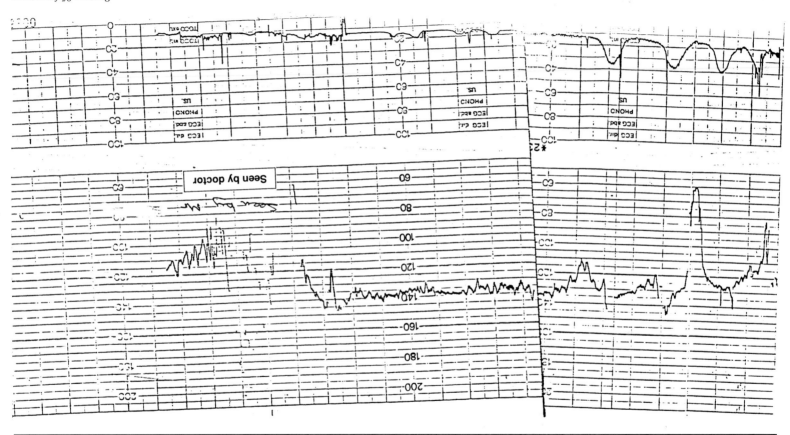

See page 85 for outcome

# Outcome

**23:13   Intrauterine death**

No partogram was kept.

A partogram is useful even when there has been an intrauterine death, as it is just as essential to monitor maternal well-being, fluid balance (particularly if oxytocin is used) and progress of labour, as obstructed labour and uterine rupture may still occur.

**10.1**
The CTG was completely unreactive with a baseline bradycardia of 110 bpm (remember at this gestation a higher rate is expected).

**10.2**
This was followed by unprovoked decelerations before the rate fell and then stopped completely.

Labour was induced with vaginal prostaglandins, and proceeded uneventfully.

Postmortem: male baby, 1.39 kg (light for gestation); large right atrium, but no other cardiac abnormality. Uteroplacental ischaemia and placental infarction.

No precise cause was found for the death of this baby. The cardiac anomaly is unlikely to be responsible for the fetal compromise but may be secondary to a maternal insult, such as a viral infection. Alternatively, the cardiomegaly may have been a reflection of intrauterine growth retardation and fetal anaemia. Had the baby been delivered earlier it may have experienced severe problems in the perinatal period, but in retrospect delivery should indeed have been expedited once the CTG became 'decelerative' (see Case 6, page 49), especially as the fetal blood sampling and Doppler studies were abnormal.

# Clinical points

## Cordocentesis

This procedure is only performed in specialist centres and involves the sampling of fetal blood from the umbilical cord, via an ultrasound-guided needle. Cordocentesis may be used to look for chromosomal abnormalities and fetal anaemia (as in rhesus isoimmunization). In addition, blood gases and pH may be measured, and this has been promoted for cases in which there is suspected fetal compromise and uncertainty as to how soon to organize delivery. There is still some debate about the effect of this invasive procedure on neonatal outcome.

## The biophysical profile

Each of the five parameters that are measured in the biophysical profile (BPP) are scored from 0 to 2, so that a maximum of 10 points equates with a good fetal outcome. The test should be performed within 2 hours of a meal, when fetal movements are maximal, and at least 2 hours after the last cigarette (although hopefully the mother will have stopped smoking long ago!). A score of 10 is achieved if the following criteria are met:

1. **CTG**: at least two accelerations of 15 bpm and 15 seconds duration in 20 minutes.
2. **Fetal breathing**: at least one episode of 30 seconds breathing in 30 minutes.
3. **Movements**: three separate limb or trunk movements in 30 minutes.
4. **Fetal tone**: one episode of extension/flexion in 30 minutes.
5. **Liquor volume**: a pocket of greater than 1 cm × 1 cm.

A score of 4 or less warrants immediate delivery (perinatal mortality is 10% if the BPP score is 4, and 60% if it is 0). A score of less than 6 is worrying, especially if liquor volume is reduced; if the baby is mature, delivery should be considered. A score of 8 indicates the need for a repeat test in 2–3 days and a score of 10 suggests a perinatal mortality of less than 1/1000 over the following week.

An additional advantage of the BPP is the opportunity to check for fetal anomalies. The test is difficult to interpret under 28 weeks' gestation as the CTG is often unreactive and fetal limb and breathing movements infrequent. The fetus breathes 50% of the time at term, yet may be quiescent for up to 2 hours. However, generally the BPP can be completed in 20 minutes, as an active baby may only require 10 minutes for the CTG and 10 for the scan. Equal weight is given to the five variables, although the best predictors of fetal well-being are movement, tone and liquor volume. The assessment of all these factors reduces unnecessary intervention for one abnormal parameter.

*Cross references:* **Antenatal monitoring** *pages 45, 49, 59, 71, 81* **The partogram** *pages 17, 23, 85*

# CASE 11

22-year Indian, married, cashier

G2 P1
1987    NVD 3.04 kg boy at
        39 weeks
No other past history

EDD 31.7.89 by USS

Booked at 16 weeks

---

16.7.89 38 weeks

00:30   Admitted with mild contractions
        Cephalic presentation
        Left occipito-anterior position
        Head 2/5 palpable
        Cervix 1 cm dilated

16:00   3 cm
        Spontaneous rupture of membranes

22:00   3 cm and now starting to contract

22:45   Pethidine given

24:30   Fully dilated

## 11.1

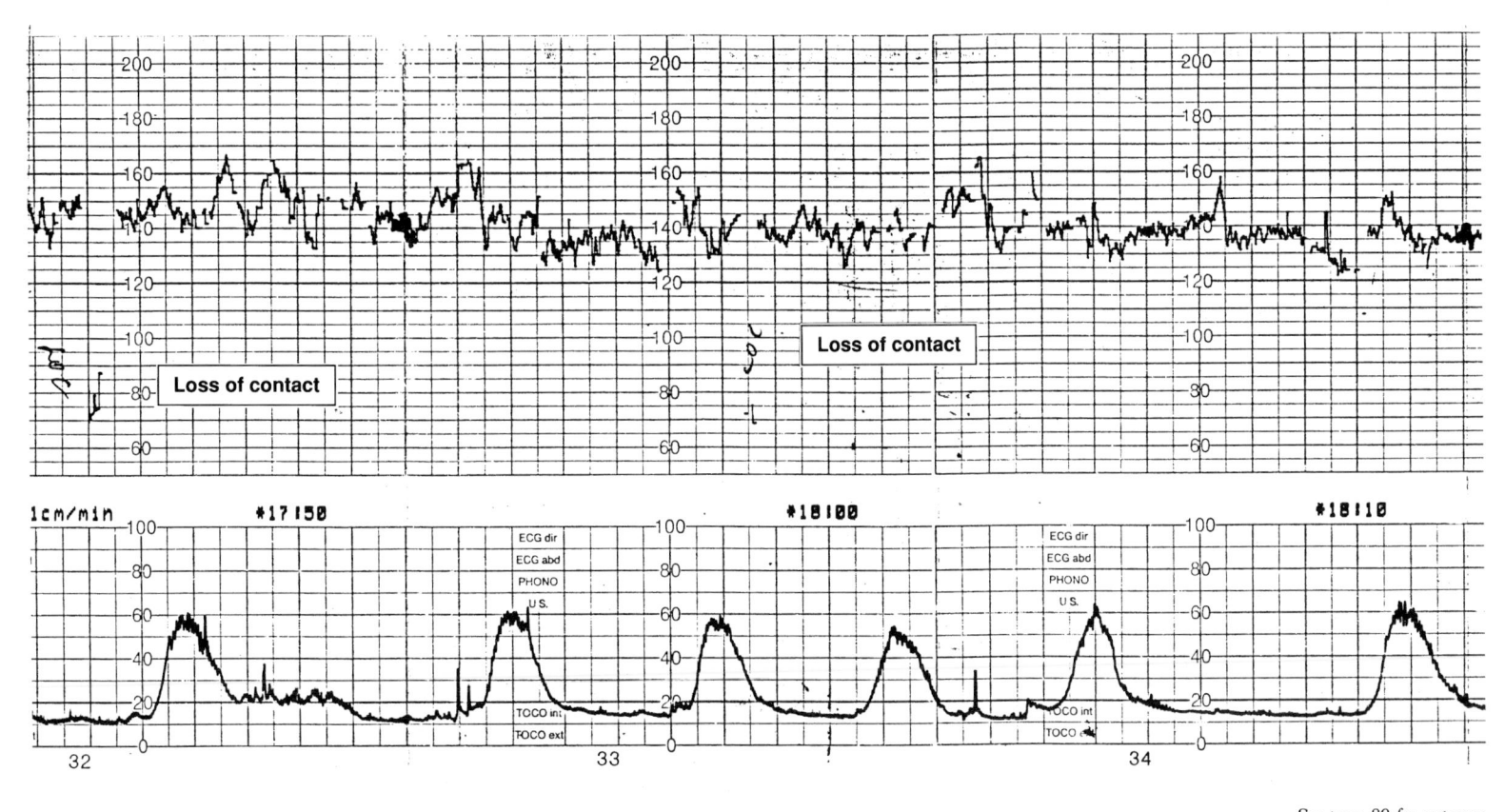

Loss of contact

Loss of contact

Loss of contact

1cm/min

*17150

*18100

*18110

*See page 89 for outcome*

# Outcome

01:06   Normal vaginal delivery
2.46 kg female
Apgars normal

No partogram was kept.

Once the labour started progress
was rapid.

**11.1**
The CTG shows a reactive trace
with a baseline of 140 bpm.

# Clinical points

## MONITORING IN LOW-RISK PREGNANCIES

With such a reactive trace and no risk factors, continuous CTG monitoring is not necessary. A CTG on admission to the labour ward is important, even in low-risk cases, as intrapartum fetal distress often reflects events that may have occurred unnoticed before labour (for example, uteroplacental insufficiency). Provided this admission CTG is normal for a period of 20 minutes, the recording may be discontinued and the labouring mother allowed to mobilize or assume her position of greatest comfort.

It is then essential intermittently to auscultate the fetal heart, every 15–20 minutes, both during and after uterine contractions. Either a Pinard stethoscope or an audible electronic device (e.g. Sonicaid)

may be used; the latter is preferable as it avoids confusing the fetal heart for the souffle of the uterine vessels, it is reassuring for the parents to hear the heart beat and it is also less uncomfortable.

In low-risk cases the only advantage of the CTG is as a 'printed record'. The potential disadvantage is that continuous monitoring may provide a false sense of security and result in too infrequent observations of the trace, which is then of less benefit than efficient intermittent auscultation. Several recent studies have indeed indicated that, provided a problem is promptly recognized, the actual method of monitoring is of little importance.

## CRITERIA FOR CONTINUOUS MONITORING

Continuous monitoring is best reserved for labours which cease to be 'physiological'. This includes labours that have been induced, augmented or are prolonged, also those associated with meconium staining, epidural analgesia, multiple fetuses, malpresentations and if there is antepartum concern about fetal well-being (for example, intrauterine growth retardation).

Cross references: **Maternal attitudes to fetal monitoring** page 109

# CASE 12

29-year, married, secretary

Primigravida
Took 5 years trying to conceive
No past history
Smoker: 15/day

LMP 10.9.89—EDD 17.6.90
Booked 14 weeks
Shared care

Uneventful pregnancy

30.6.90 42 weeks

05:15    Admitted contracting since 03:00
           Cephalic presentation
           Left occipito-anterior position
           Head 2/5 palpable abdominally
           Cervix admits 'fingertip'
           Contractions weak

15:00    Now contracting regularly
           3 cm dilated
           Amniotomy (artificial rupture of
           membranes), clear liquor
           Epidural requested

19:00    4–5 cm
           Oxytocin infusion suggested (started at 20:00)

22:00    5 cm
           Oxytocin increased

02:05    Fully dilated
           Occipito-anterior (OA) position
           Head not palpable abdominally

# 12.1

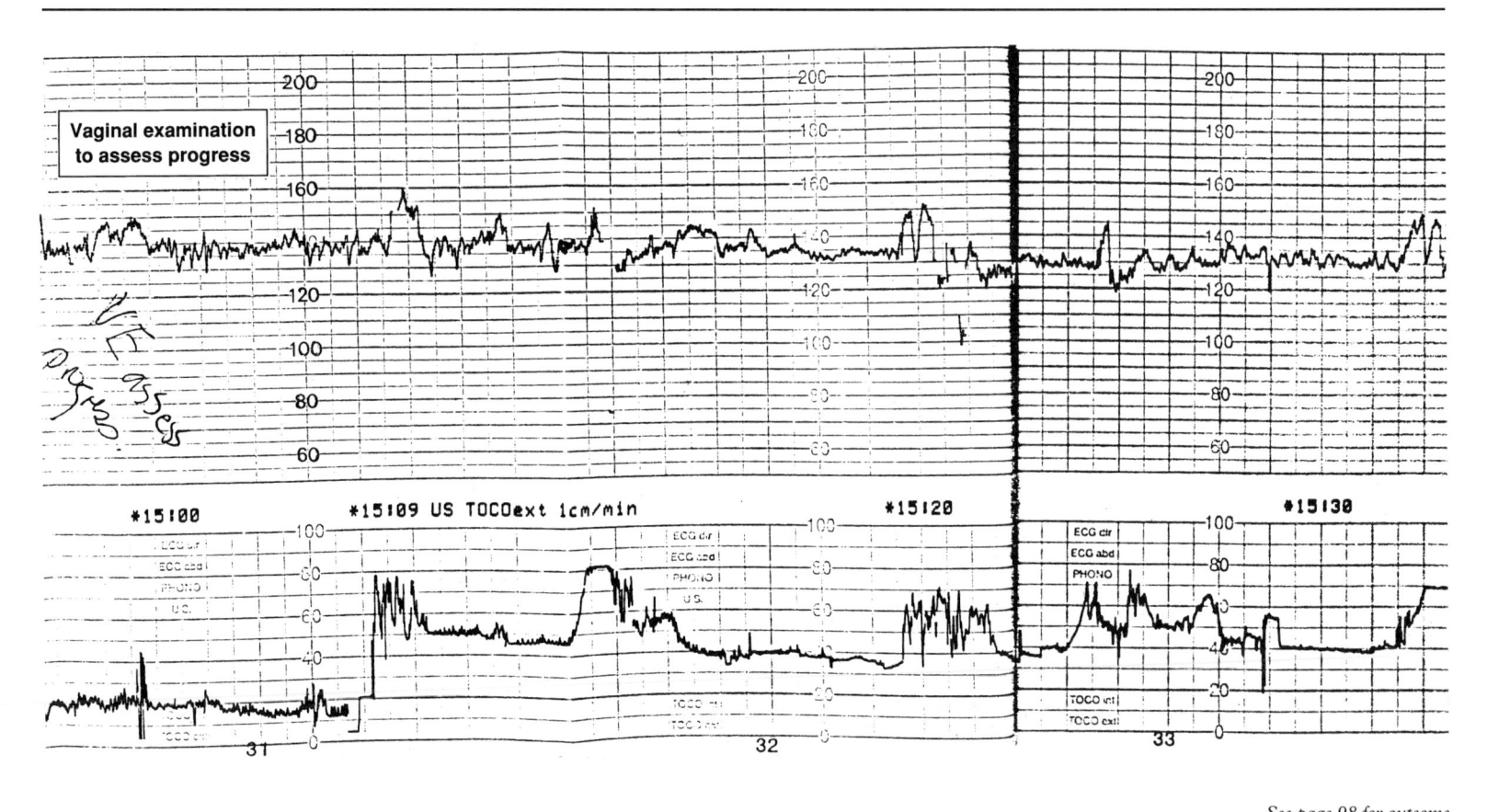

*See page 98 for outcome*

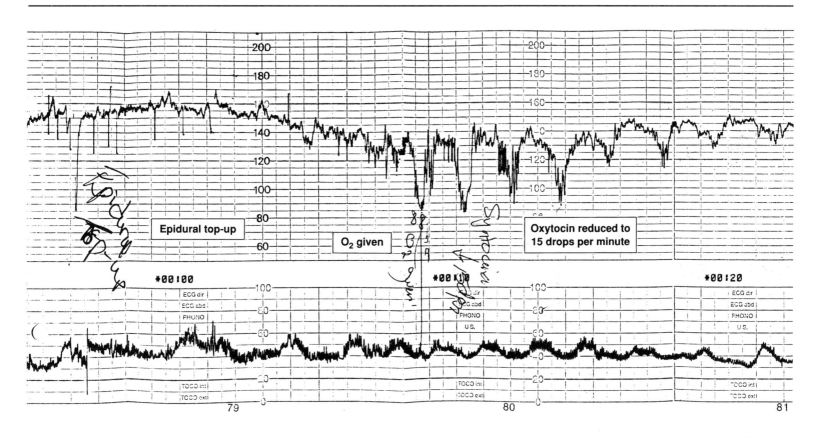

Epidural top-up

$O_2$ given

Oxytocin reduced to
15 drops per minute

*00¦00

*00¦10

*00¦20

79

80

81

*See page 98 for outcome*

# 12.3

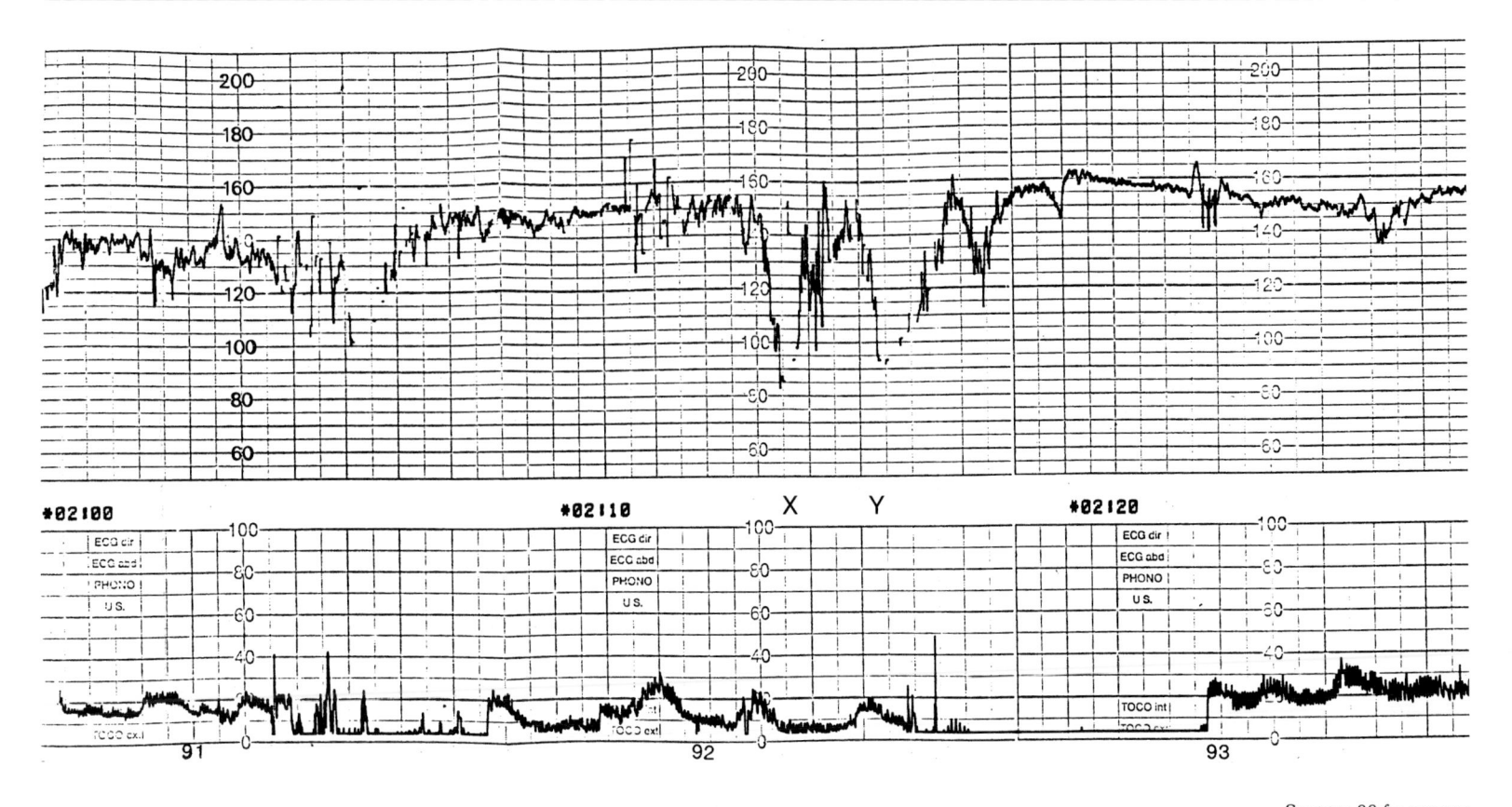

*See page 98 for outcome*

# 12.4

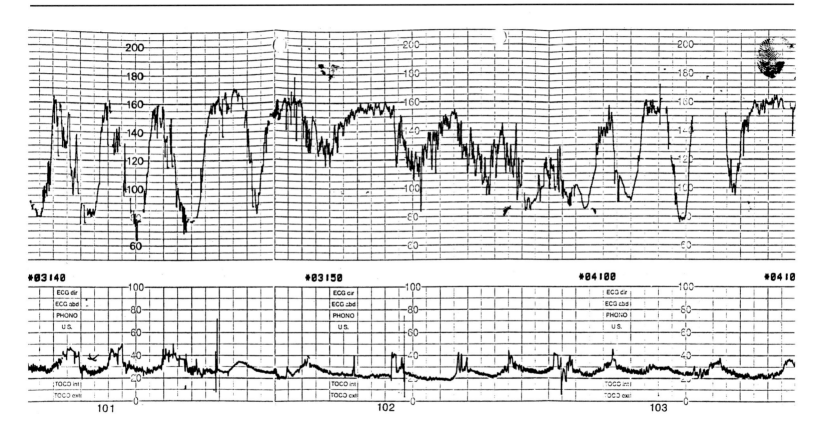

*See page 98 for outcome*

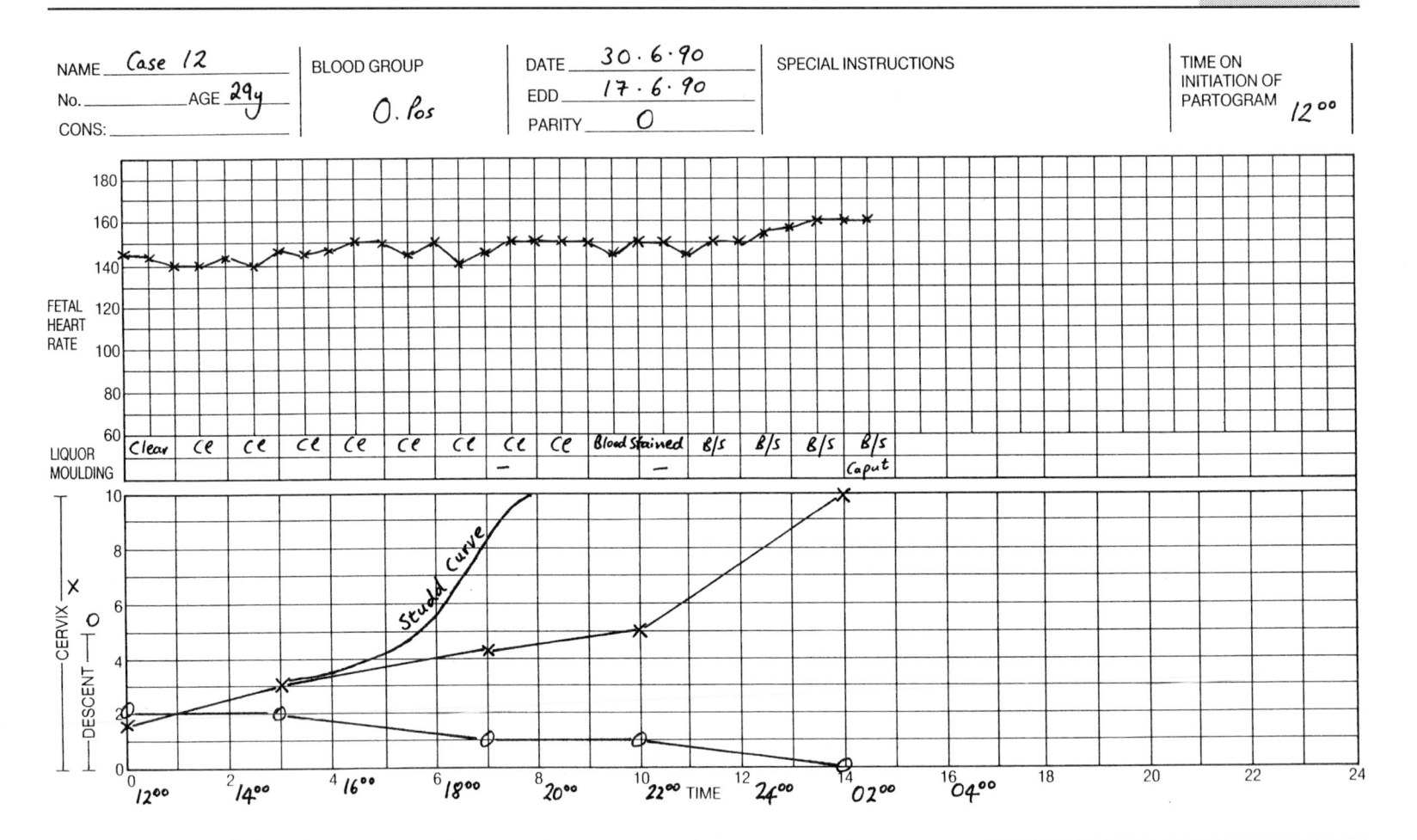

NAME _Case 12_

No. _____ AGE **29y**

CONS: _____

BLOOD GROUP

O. Pos

DATE ___30·6·90___

EDD ___17·6·90___

PARITY ___0___

SPECIAL INSTRUCTIONS

TIME ON
INITIATION OF
PARTOGRAM   12°°

FETAL HEART RATE

180
160
140
120
100
80
60

LIQUOR MOULDING

| Clear | Ce | Ce | Ce | Ce | Ce | Ce | Ce | Ce | Blood Stained | B/s | B/s | B/s | B/s |
| | | | | | | | − | | − | | | | Caput |

CERVIX ✗
DESCENT ○

10
8
6
4
2
0

Studd Curve

TIME

12°°  14°°  16°°  18°°  20°°  22°°  24°°  02°°  04°°

0  2  4  6  8  10  12  14  16  18  20  22  24

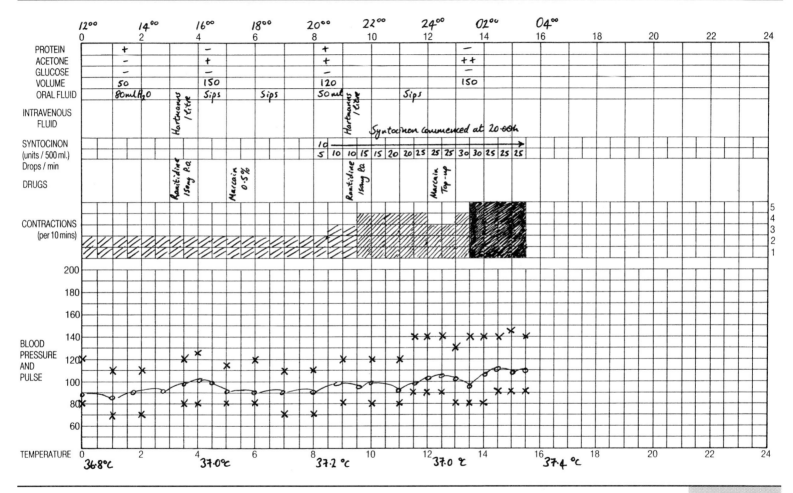

# Outcome

03:30   Neville–Barnes forceps delivery
        Occipito-anterior position
        3.175 kg male
        Apgars 8/1 10/5

The partogram clearly charts the progress of labour. Oxytocin was started for a primary dysfunctional labour after which progress was normal.

**12.1**
Baseline 140 bpm, good variability and accelerations with uterine activity.

**12.2**
The straight vertical lines at the beginning of the trace are artefactual (i.e. due to fluctuations in the machine or maternal movements rather than having any real significance). There is good variability and Type 2 decelerations with quick recovery and small accelerations, suggesting that fetal compromise is minimal.

**12.3**
Baseline has risen slightly. X and Y are Type 2 decelerations. The contraction belt is not placed properly and so not recording very well.

**12.4**
Baseline now 160 bpm, appears reactive, but the decelerations are all Type 2 and deeper. As the patient was fully dilated a forceps delivery was performed.

# Clinical points

## EPIDURALS

Most obstetricians would agree that continuous fetal monitoring is essential when using this form of analgesia. The reasons are twofold: firstly, to monitor the possible effects of the epidural on the fetal heart rate, and also because the epidural may have been required for a labour that is already in a higher risk category. Epidural top-ups may cause maternal hypotension and hence uterine hypoperfusion, resulting in a temporary fetal bradycardia. This can be minimized by pre-loading the mother with intravenous fluids and avoiding supine hypotension, by tilting the bed laterally at a 45° angle (this prevents aortocaval compression of the uterus). Sometimes the anaesthetist has to give ephedrine to raise the blood pressure.

Epidurals should not affect the rate of progress of the first stage of labour—but of course they are often given to women experiencing a difficult labour, and hence incorrectly blamed for the problems!

As to its effect on the second stage, an epidural inhibits the sensation of the bearing-down reflex and depresses the tone of the pelvic floor musculature. Thus an effective epidural may prolong the second stage of labour and delay rotation of the fetal head. Starting oxytocin in the second stage has been found to reduce the need for an instrumental delivery, particularly if the fetal head is already in the occipito-anterior position.

## INSTRUMENTAL DELIVERY

The reasons for performing an instrumental (forceps or ventouse) delivery range from an elective forceps delivery (e.g. medical reasons for avoiding maternal effort in the second stage, or for the after-coming head in a breech) to expediting delivery when there is fetal distress or maternal exhaustion. It is essential to know the position and station of the fetal head (see Case 22, page 175).

If there is fetal distress and no mechanical obstruction to delivery, then either an 'outlet' forceps delivery or ventouse extraction may swiftly be performed. However, before proceeding with a rotational delivery in the presence of apparent fetal distress on the CTG, one should have excluded acidosis by sampling the fetal scalp blood (see Case 13, page 108).

*Cross references:* **Epidurals** *pages 33, 40*

# CASE 13

23-year Irish, single, unemployed

G2 P0 +1 (TOP)
No other history

EDD 4.5.90
Booked at 20 weeks

Uneventful pregnancy

| | |
|---|---|
| 2.5.90 | 39+ weeks<br>Admitted with spontaneous rupture of membranes<br>Cephalic presentation<br>Occipito-posterior position<br>Head 2/5 palpable |
| 00:20 | Cervix 4–5 cm dilated |
| 03:10 | Pethidine |
| 07:20 | 4 cm<br>Epidural then oxytocin |
| 10:15 | 5–6 cm<br>Right occipito-posterior position<br>Oxytocin not started until now |
| 11:25 | Regular strong contractions |
| 12:45 | Fully dilated<br>Head not palpable abdominally<br>Right occipito-transverse position |

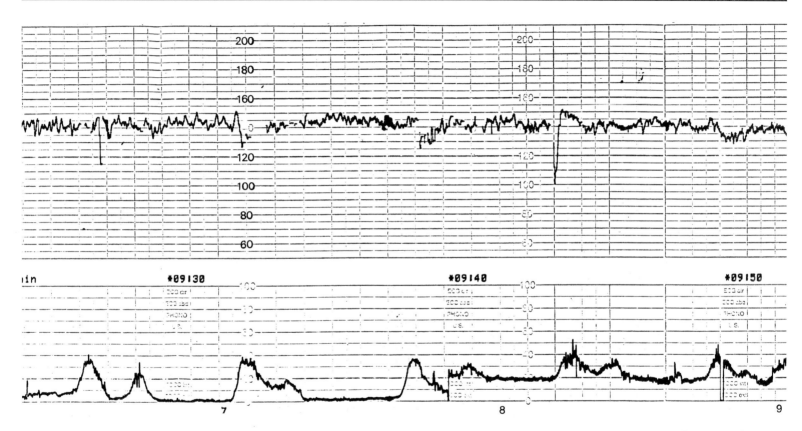

*See page 108 for outcome*

# 13.2

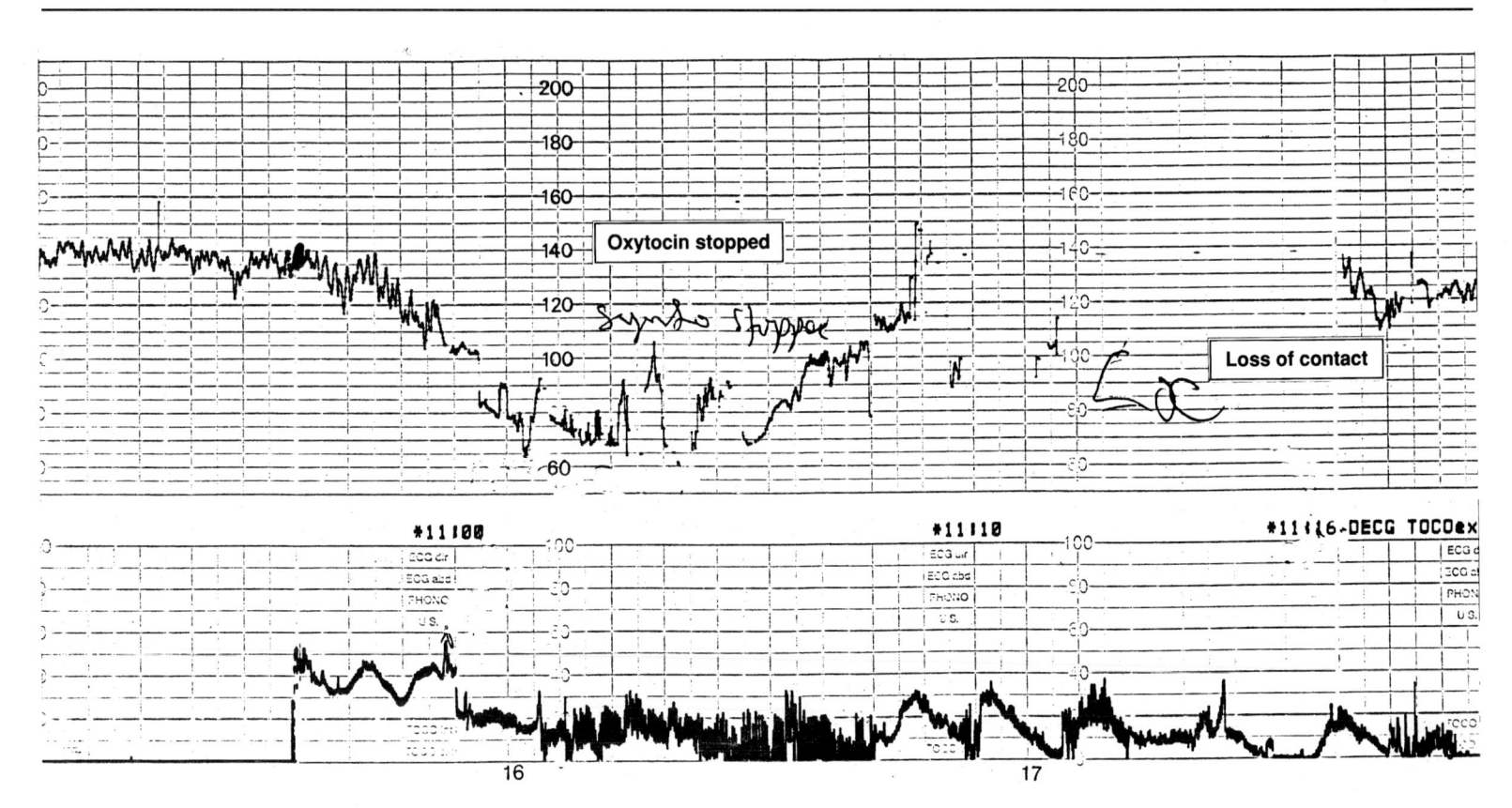

See page 108 for outcome

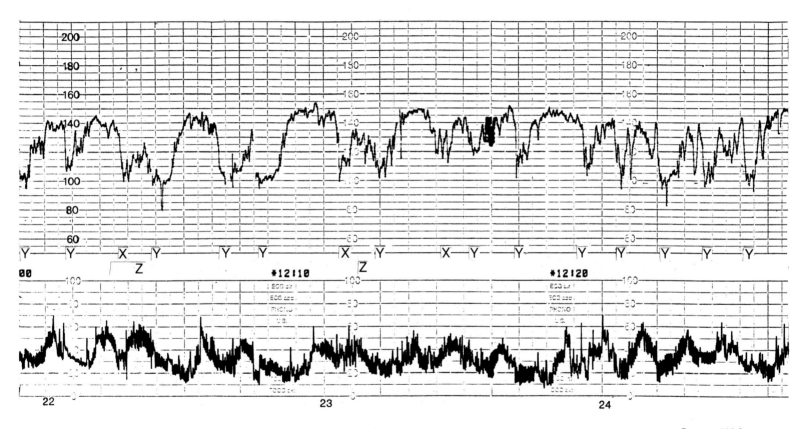

*See page 108 for outcome*

# 13.4

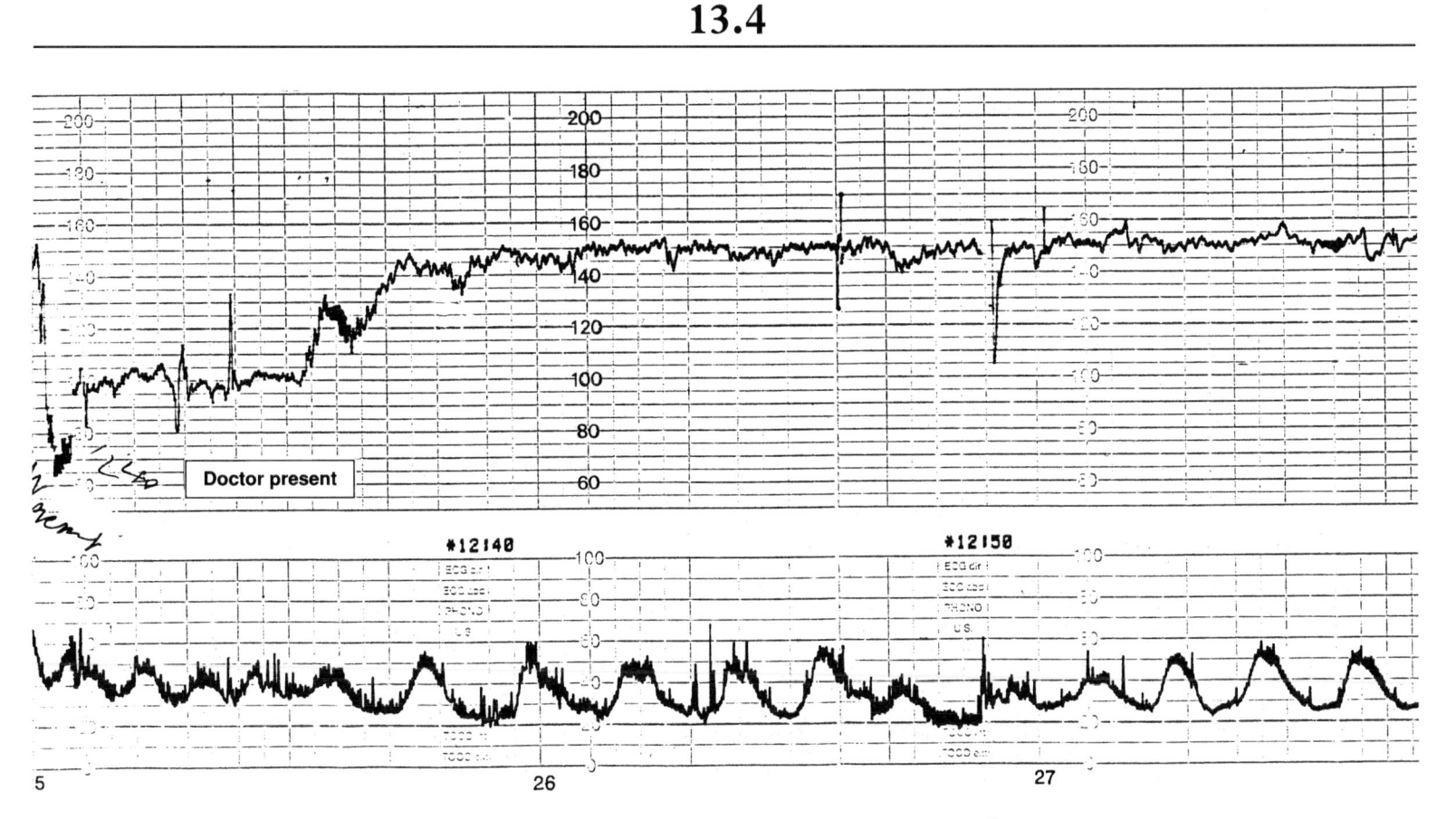

**Doctor present**

*See page 108 for outcome*

# 13.5

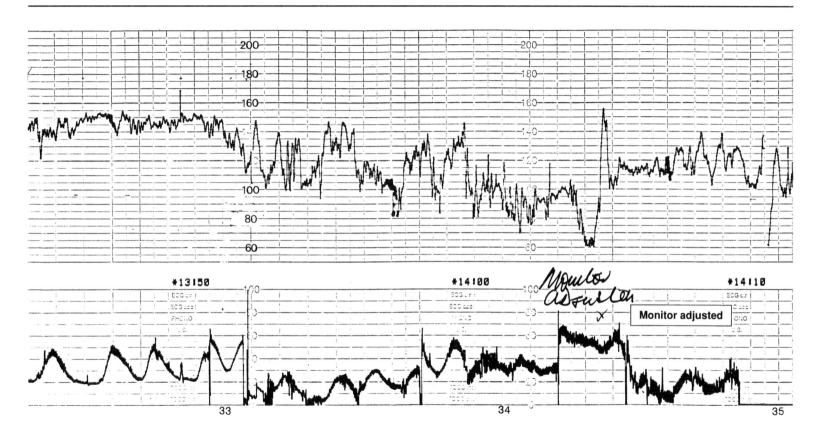

*See page 108 for outcome*

**CASE 13**

NAME _Case 13_

No. _____ AGE _23y_

CONS: _____

BLOOD GROUP

_B +_

DATE _2.5.90_

EDD _4.5.90_

PARITY _O +1_

SPECIAL INSTRUCTIONS

TIME ON
INITIATION OF
PARTOGRAM _07∞h_

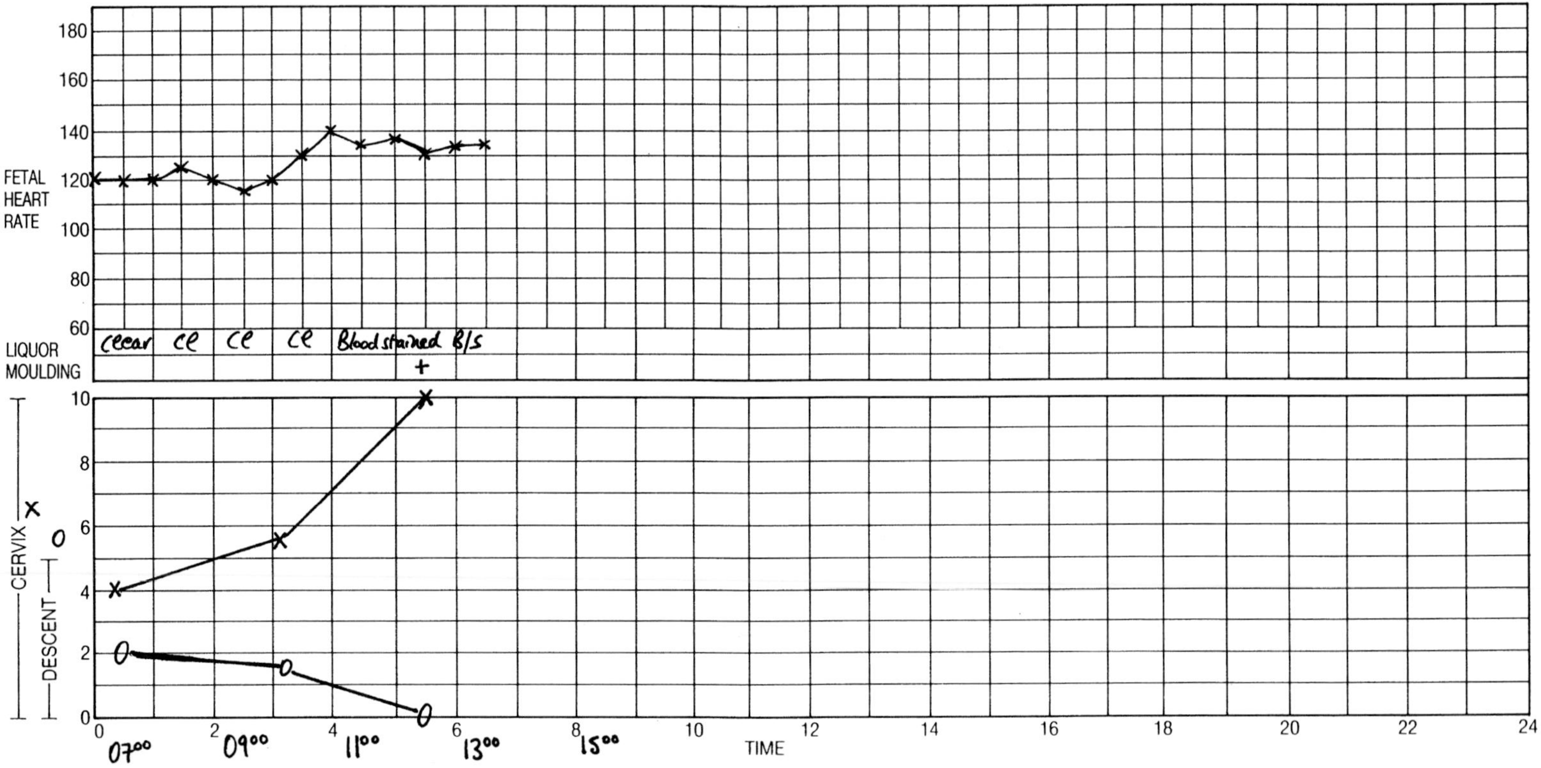

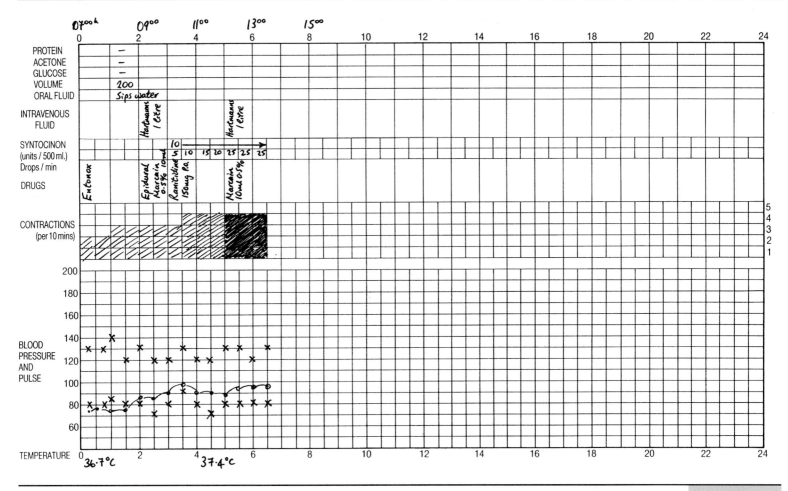

# Outcome

13:45   Kielland's forceps delivery
        3.24 kg male
        Apgars 9/1 10/5

The partogram was started too late; too long a time was left between the first and second vaginal examination, and there was no progress. This was a primary dysfunctional labour and so oxytocin was started.

**13.1**
Good variability, baseline 140–150 bpm. No accelerations; contractions coupling.

**13.2**
Oxytocin has now been started, there was a prolonged deceleration and loss of contact—a fetal scalp electrode really should be used in every woman with an epidural.

**13.3**
With good variability there are variable decelerations (X Type 1, Y Type 2), and some prolonged 'W'-shaped decelerations without full recovery to the baseline (Z).

**13.4**
After a prolonged bradycardia there is now reduced variability at a rate of 150 bpm.

In view of the transverse position of the fetal head it was decided to wait for rotation before pushing.

**13.5**
Variability has improved, but the baseline then falls with larger swings in rate. There was no rotation after an hour in second stage with good contractions. Kielland's rotational delivery was performed. Ideally fetal blood sampling should have been performed beforehand. The infant was in a good condition and the decelerations were probably due to relative cephalopelvic disproportion secondary to the transverse position.

# Clinical points

It is essential that a mother understands the reasons for wishing to monitor her baby and also the results, whether good or bad (as often only bad results are explained, leaving a couple to worry unnecessarily when things are alright). It helps if the reasons for, and methods of, monitoring are introduced during antenatal classes so that the parents have an idea of what to expect on the labour ward. Some women find the CTG reassuring, whilst others become alarmed by changes in heart rate which may be normal. If there is loss of contact, especially if the midwife has left the room, many parents think that the baby's heart itself has stopped. Similarly, a deceleration to 60 bpm appears to the untrained eye to be 0 bpm, as this is the bottom of the recording, and so it is important to explain exactly what is being seen.

Some women like to hear the fetal heart beat and feel happier being continuously monitored. Others find the elastic belts uncomfortable and restrictive and sometimes object to any monitoring at all. If one is sympathetic to the wishes of the mother, most will be happy with a baseline CTG in early labour and will then permit intermittent auscultation. This should be done whenever possible with an electronic device so that the parents may hear the baby's heart beat.

If continuous monitoring is felt to be necessary, a careful explanation results in the consent of most women. One should always ask before applying a scalp electrode, as great alarm and unhappiness may result if it is attached without prior knowledge. Most mothers are concerned about possible harm to their baby and they should be reassured that there is little risk of serious complications (provided the fontanelles are avoided) and that scalp electrodes do not cause maternal infection. The ultimate aim of labour is a safe outcome for both mother and baby. Whilst this does require monitoring to a degree that varies with each individual clinical situation, usually it should be possible to care for the parents in a calm and reassuring manner, without them feeling overwhelmed by technology.

*Cross references:* **Epidurals** *pages 33, 40, 99* **The partogram** *pages 17, 23, 85* **Monitoring in labour** *page 90* **The fetal scalp electrode** *page 151*

# CASE 14

18-year single, unemployed

Primigravida
No past history

EDD 9.3.90

Booked late at 27 weeks

Uneventful pregnancy

1.3.90   Admitted for assessment with polyhydramnios
Normal glucose tolerance test

21.3.90 41+ weeks
Readmitted contracting
Head 4/5 palpable

19:00   Cervix 2–3 cm dilated

22:40   4 cm
Amniotomy, liquor +++
Cord prolapse

# 14.1

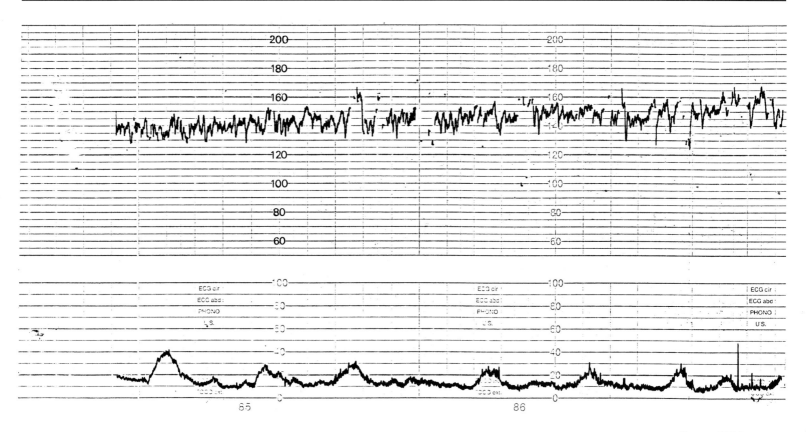

*See page 113 for outcome*

## 14.2

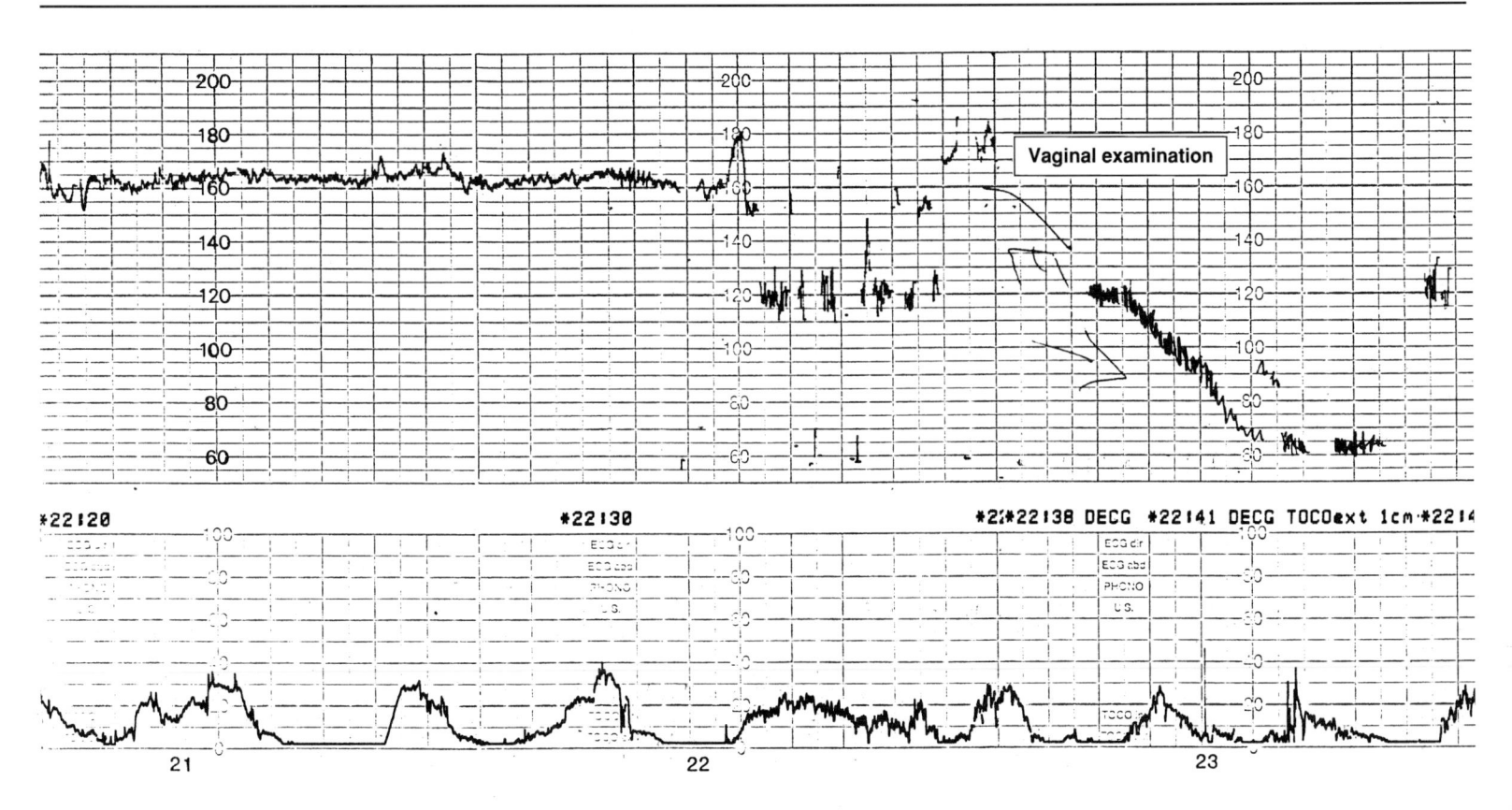

Vaginal examination

*See page 113 for outcome*

# Outcome

22:50   Emergency caesarean section
        3.30 kg female
        Apgars 8/1 8/5 9/10

No partogram was kept!

**14.1**
Good variability with a baseline of
140–150 bpm.

**14.2**
The heart rate plummets with amniotomy
and the umbilical cord prolapses.

# Clinical points

## AMNIOTOMY WITH POLYHYDRAMNIOS

Cord prolapse should have been predicted in this case, as there was both poly-hydramnios and a high head. If amniotomy was felt to be essential, appropriate precautions should have been taken. The patient should have been prepared for a caesarean section, with an epidural and intravenous line sited, the anaesthetist and paediatrician present and the procedure performed in the operating theatre.

It has been suggested that a controlled release of amniotic fluid may be achieved by piercing the membranes with a needle and restricting the flow with a strategically placed finger, but in reality the liquor usually gushes out. Alternatively, amniocentesis prior to amniotomy enables much of the fluid to be withdrawn. If the woman is in labour it is best to perform the amniotomy during a contraction, so that the head is encouraged to enter the pelvis at the same time.

## CORD PROLAPSE

When the umbilical cord prolapses the baby should be delivered immediately, and by caesarean section, unless the cervix is fully dilated and an easy instrumental delivery is anticipated. Many methods have been described to take the pressure off the cord, but the easiest approach is to keep a hand inside the vagina (to displace the head) and either raise the foot of the bed or place the mother in the knee–elbow position. The midwife's/doctor's hand should be removed only when the baby has been delivered.

# CASE 15

30-year housewife

G3 P2

1986    Kielland's forceps
        delivery, 3.3 kg girl
1989    NVD 2.65 kg boy

No other history

EDD 7.4.90

Booked 15 weeks
Shared care

Breech presentation from
38 weeks

Pelvimetry—inlet   13.0 cm
          —outlet 11.1 cm

Scan estimated weight 3.57 kg,
frank breech

19.4.90 41+ weeks

09:00    Admitted in labour
         Cervix 6 cm dilated
         Amniotomy, clear liquor
         Epidural sited
         Fetal scalp electrode applied

15:00    No progress after 6 hours

# 15.1

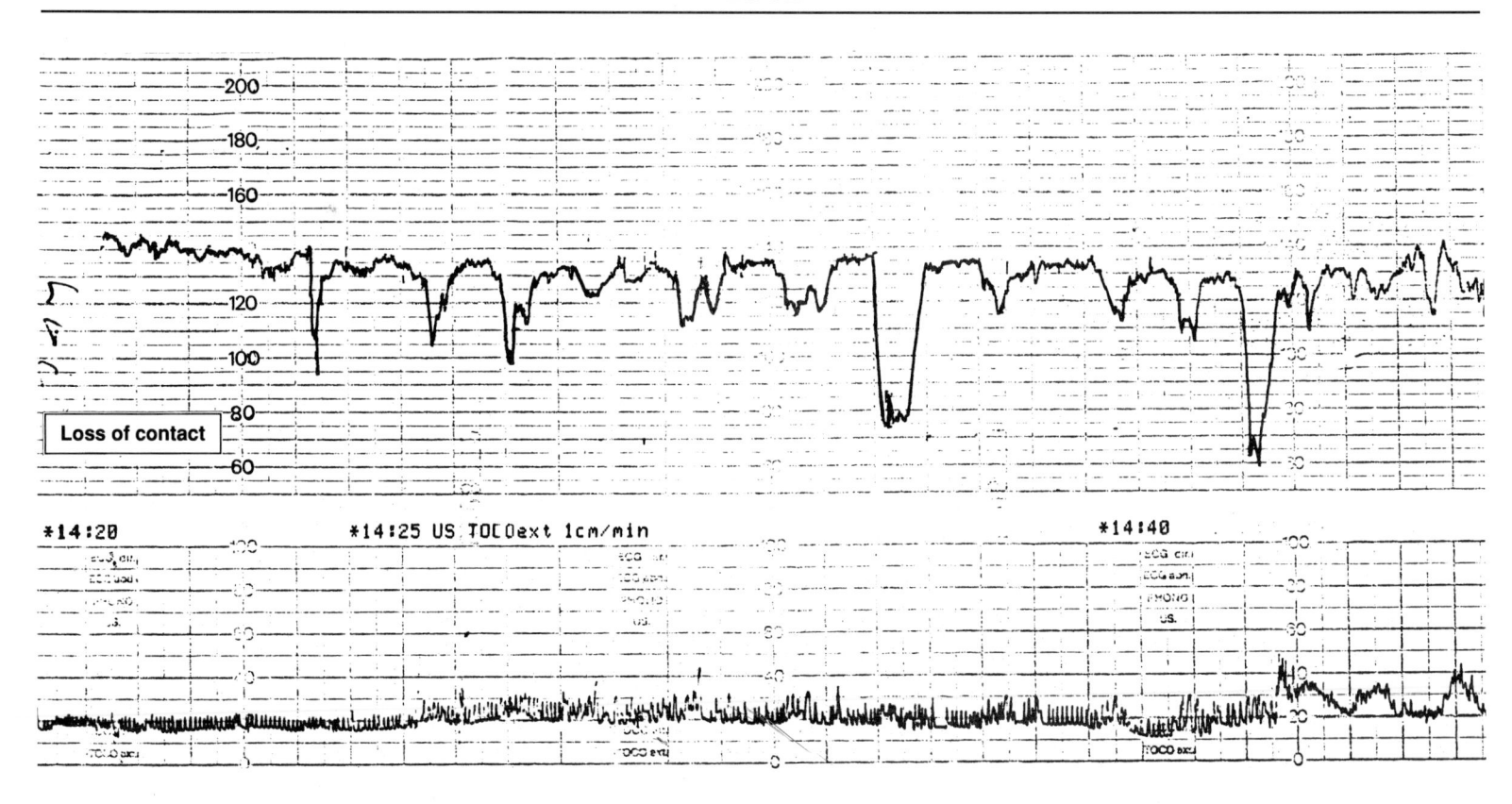

Loss of contact

*14:20      *14:25 US TOCOext 1cm/min      *14:40

*See page 117 for outcome*

# Outcome

15:30    Emergency caesarean section
3.62 kg male
Apgars normal
No cord entanglement

No partogram was kept.

The contraction belt was badly placed and therefore did not give any information about uterine activity.

**15.1**
The baseline is 130 bpm, there are several decelerations.

Caesarean section was necessary as most obstetricians agree that it is inappropriate to augment a breech labour with oxytocin. Note also that X-ray pelvimetry serves only as a guide to allowing labour when there is a breech presentation; the type of breech (i.e. flexed or extended), together with the estimated weight of the baby, should also be considered. Pelvimetry alone is a poor predictor for the outcome of labour.

# Clinical points

## BREECH PRESENTATION

Decelerations in a breech are usually significant as there is obviously not the head compression seen with a cephalic presentation. They may be due to cord compression, and one should always remember that the risk of cord prolapse is increased when there is a malpresentation. Sometimes the cord may lie trapped between the presenting part and the cervix and so not be immediately noticable as a complete prolapse.

In the above case a caesarean section was performed for failure of progress in labour and the baby was healthy. A blood sample may be taken from a breech although one should be careful not to make a large cut, as the skin is more easily damaged, and, unlike the scalp, will not later be covered with hair.

## MECONIUM: 2

Meconium staining of the liquor is a normal occurrence in breech presentations. It is coloured green by bile acids. Meconium may also be passed normally in about 20% of babies presenting by the head; in about 10% it is passed before labour.

Fetal diarrhoea may be a result of either infection or thyrotoxicosis. The passage of meconium prior to 34 weeks gestation is pathological and suggests infection with *Listeria*.

*Cross references:*   **Epidurals**  *pages 33, 40, 99*   **Meconium**  *page 33*   **Cord prolapse**  *page 114*

24-year Asian housewife
Height 1.47 m

Primigravida
No past history

LMP 9.10.89—EDD 16.7.90

Booked 18 weeks

Uneventful pregnancy

| 1.7.90 | 37+ weeks |
|---|---|
| 20:45 | Spontaneously ruptured membranes for 16 hours<br>Cervix 2–3 cm dilated<br>Apyrexial |
| 23:20 | Decision taken to start oxytocin in view of prolonged rupture of membranes (ROM)<br><br>Rapid progress in labour |

# 16.1

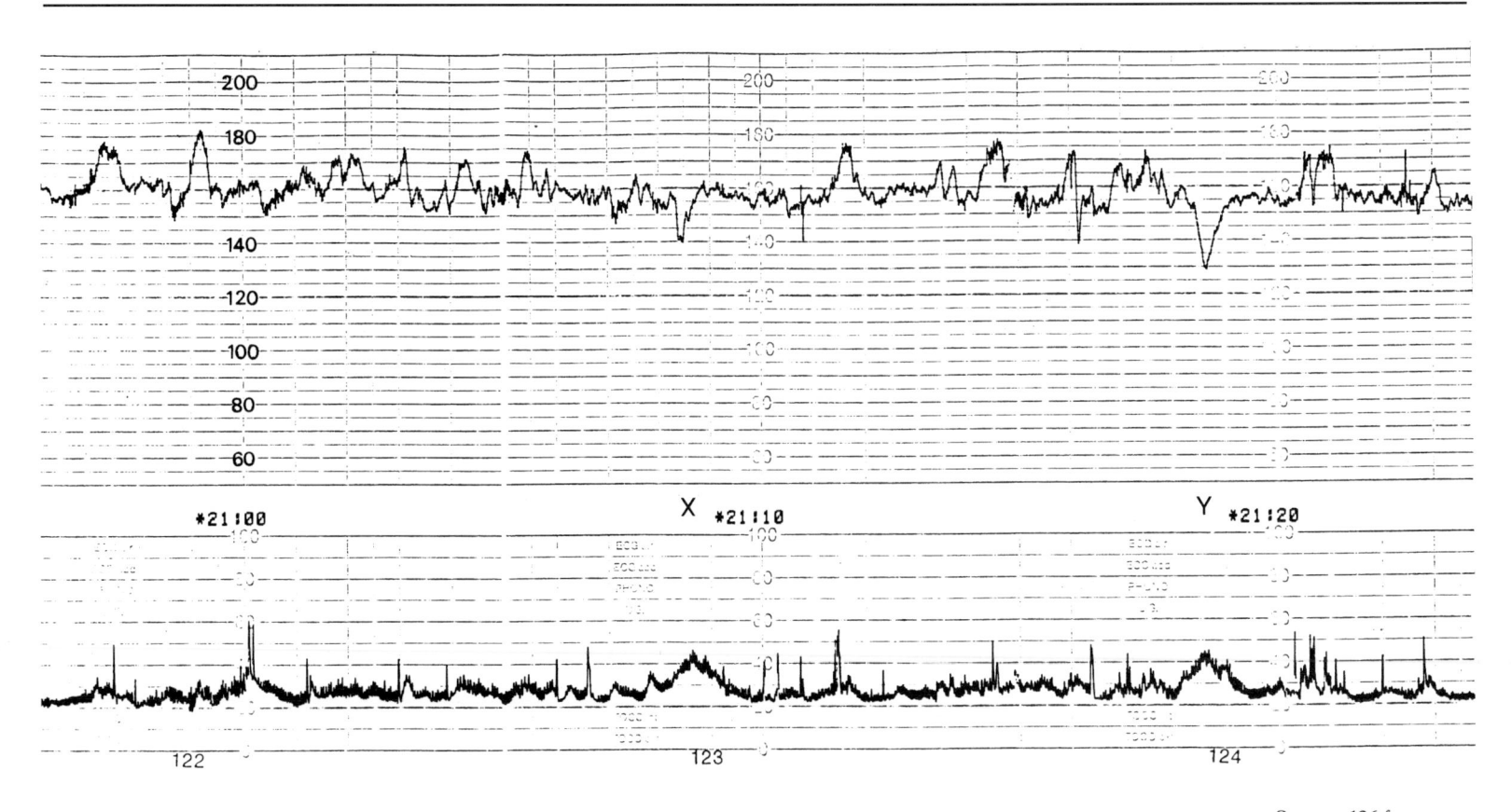

*See page 126 for outcome*

# 16.2

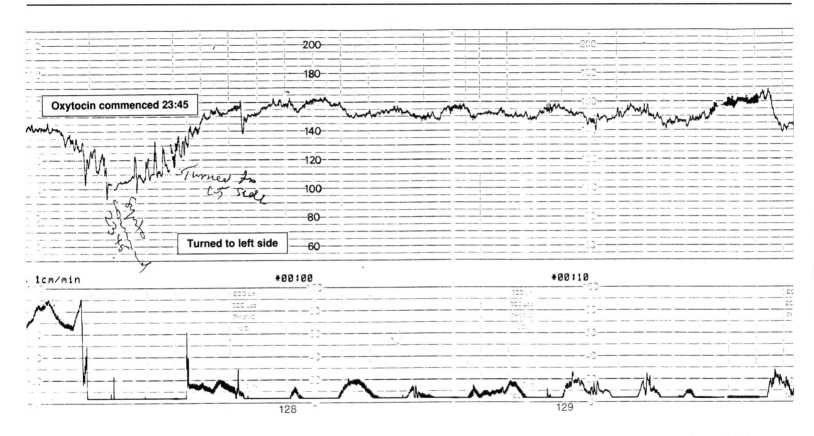

Oxytocin commenced 23:45

Turned to left side

1cm/min

*00:00

*00:10

128

129

*See page 126 for outcome*

# 16.3

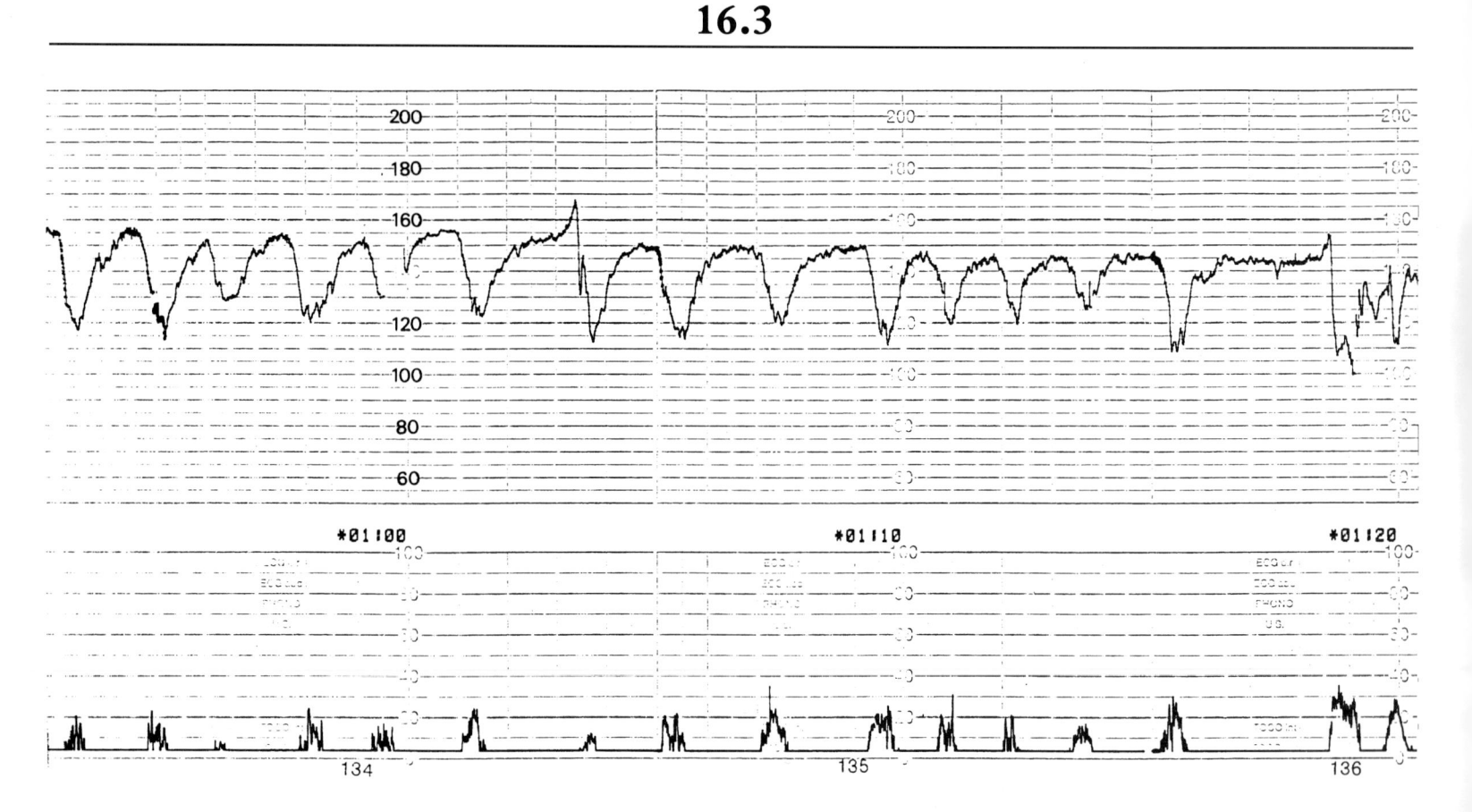

*See page 126 for outcome*

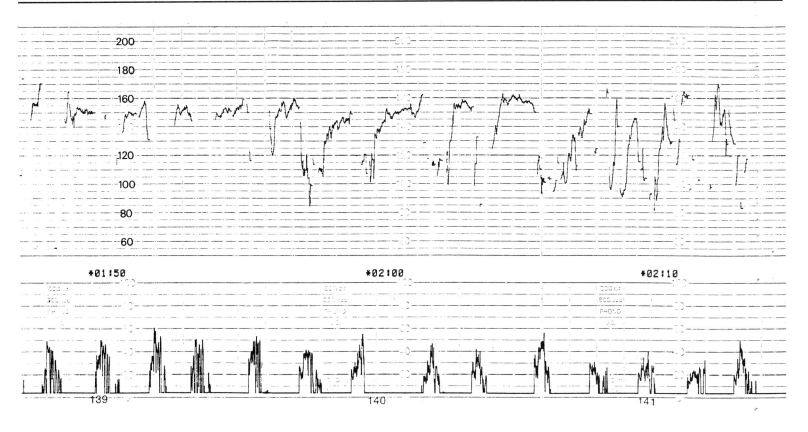

200
180
160
120
100
80
60

*01:50          *02:00          *02:10

139          140          141

*See page 126 for outcome*

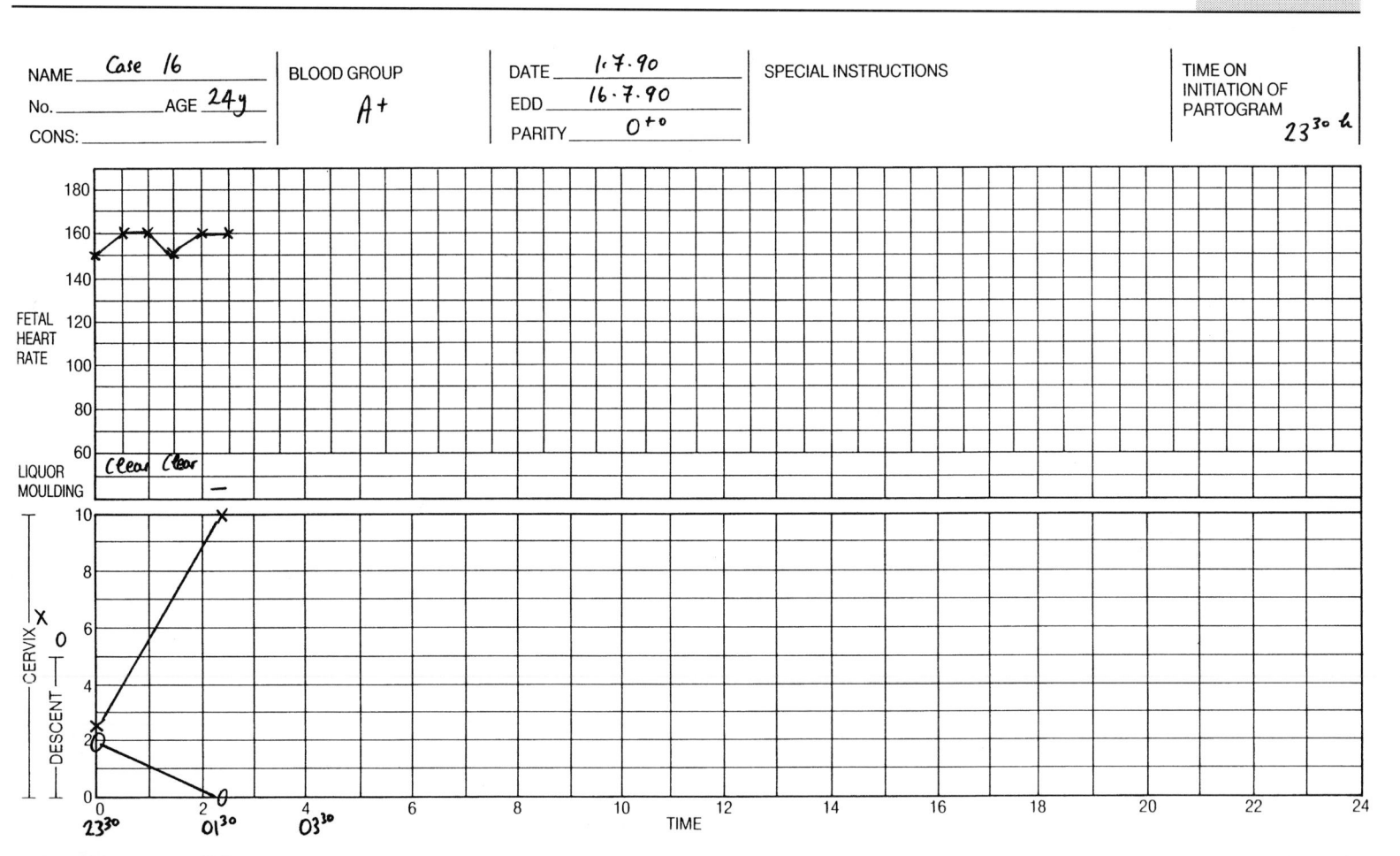

NAME _Case 16_

No. _____ AGE _24y_

CONS: _____

BLOOD GROUP

_A+_

DATE _1.7.90_

EDD _16.7.90_

PARITY _0⁺⁰_

SPECIAL INSTRUCTIONS

TIME ON
INITIATION OF
PARTOGRAM
_23³⁰ h_

FETAL HEART RATE

LIQUOR
MOULDING

CERVIX

DESCENT

TIME

Clear Clear

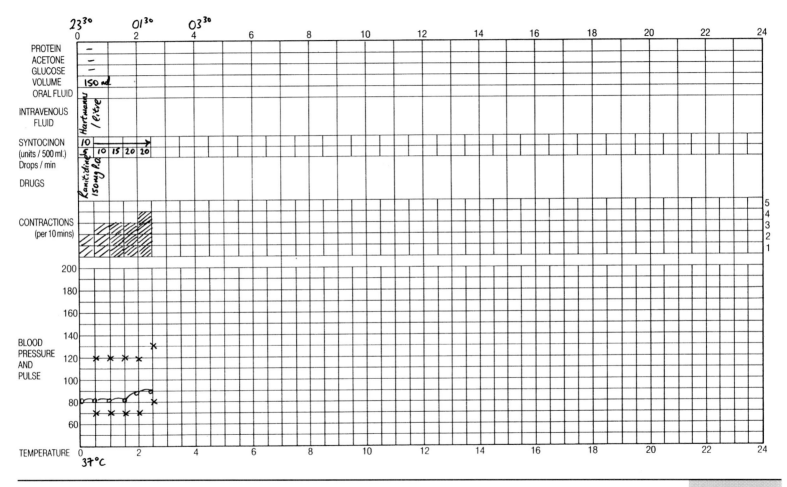

# Outcome

02:00   Spontaneous delivery
2.6 kg female
Apgars 9/1 10/5

**16.1**
Baseline 160 bpm, good variability and
accelerations. X and Y are minor Type 1
decelerations. A baseline greater than 160
in a woman with prolonged ROM may
suggest infection, particularly if there is
maternal pyrexia or tachycardia.

**16.2**
There is decreased variability here; the
prolonged deceleration appears to be
secondary to a hypertonic contraction,
which itself could have resulted from a
bolus of oxytocin (this may also cause a fall
in blood pressure, although in a dilute
solution it should have minimal effect on
the BP). Maybe a bolus was accidentally
injected at the start of the infusion.

**16.3**
The contraction belt is simply providing an
indication of when the contractions are
occurring—an external monitor will not
show the strength of contractions, only an
internal pressure transducer can do this.
All these decelerations are Type 1 with
quick recovery. Reduced variability
continues.

**16.4**
The quality of this trace is poor. If there is
any doubt about a CTG a fetal scalp
electrode should be applied. Again these
decelerations are Type 1 with recovery to a
constant baseline. If the baseline falls with
Type 1 decelerations then delivery should
be expedited (see Case 2, page 23).

# Clinical points

## EATING IN LABOUR

The stomach empties slowly in late pregnancy and a policy of fasting during labour does not hasten this process. Many women do not feel like eating but for those who are hungry, labour will be more stressful. Aspiration of stomach contents only occurs if a general anaesthetic is given, and its occurrence is minimized by the application of cricoid pressure (Sellick's manoeuvre) during induction of anaesthesia. Although it is not easy to predict those women who will have a normal delivery, it is reasonable to allow women at low risk to have a light meal during the early phase of labour. This should be of low residue and low fat content (soft fruit, fruit juices, plain biscuits).

## ANTACIDS IN LABOUR

Ranitidine was given routinely in the early part of labour, despite the short duration of labour in this case. Many labour wards have a policy of antacid administration which is aimed at minimizing the risk of pulmonary aspiration of gastric contents and the resultant pneumonitis (Mendelson's syndrome). The length of labour cannot be predicted, therefore a policy of routine 6 hourly oral ranitidine (150 mg) reduces gastric acid production. If it becomes necessary to perform an emergency caesarean section, an intramuscular injection of 50 mg ranitidine may be given, together with metoclopramide (10 mg intramuscularly), which promotes gastric emptying and 30 ml of 0.3 M sodium citrate, which is a non-particulate antacid that should neutralize any remaining gastric acid.

## PROLONGED MEMBRANE RUPTURE

Oxytocin was started for prolonged ROM—some obstetricians do this after 12 hours, some after 24 hours and others are more conservative, awaiting the spontaneous onset of labour which occurs within 48 hours in 95% of women at 'term' (i.e. past 37 weeks). As can be seen, labour progressed rapidly once the oxytocin was started.

The most important thing to remember is to keep vaginal examinations to an absolute minimum. An aseptic speculum examination should be performed to diagnose ruptured membranes, and a swab for culture can be taken at the same time. There is no need to repeat the examination until the woman is thought to be in labour.

*Cross references:* **Falling baseline** *page 23* **Intravenous fluids** *pages 175, 176*

**CASE 16**

# CASE 17

31-year Ghanian, married, canteen assistant

Primigravida
No past history

LMP 7.9.88–EDD 14.6.89

Booked 12 weeks

Pregnancy complicated by intermittent right-sided pain and scan indicated a pedunculated fibroid which was managed conservatively.

22.6.89 41 weeks

|  | |
|---|---|
| 20:00 | Admitted contracting<br>Cephalic presentation<br>Right occipito-posterior (ROP) position<br>Head 3/5 palpable<br>Cervix 1 cm dilated |
| 23:20 | 3–4 cm<br>Amniotomy, clear liquor |
| 23:50 | Pethidine |
| 02:50 | 6 cm<br>Good contractions |
| 06:00 | 6 cm<br>Clear liquor |
| 07:30 | 6 cm<br>Still ROP and no descent of head<br>CTG unsatisfactory for oxytocin |

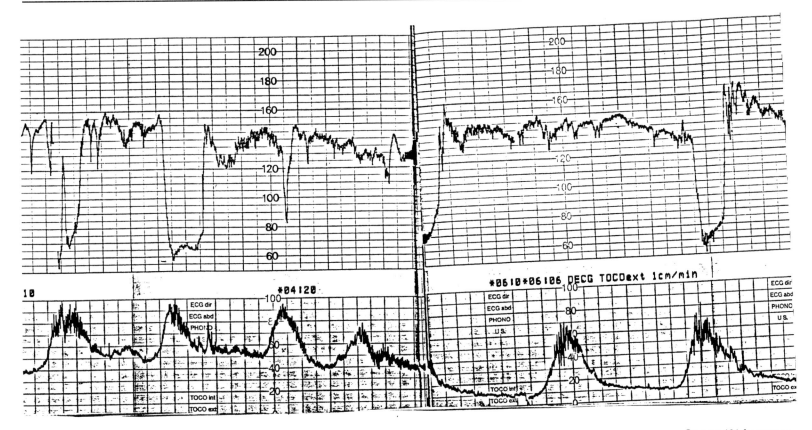

*See page 131 for outcome*

# 17.2

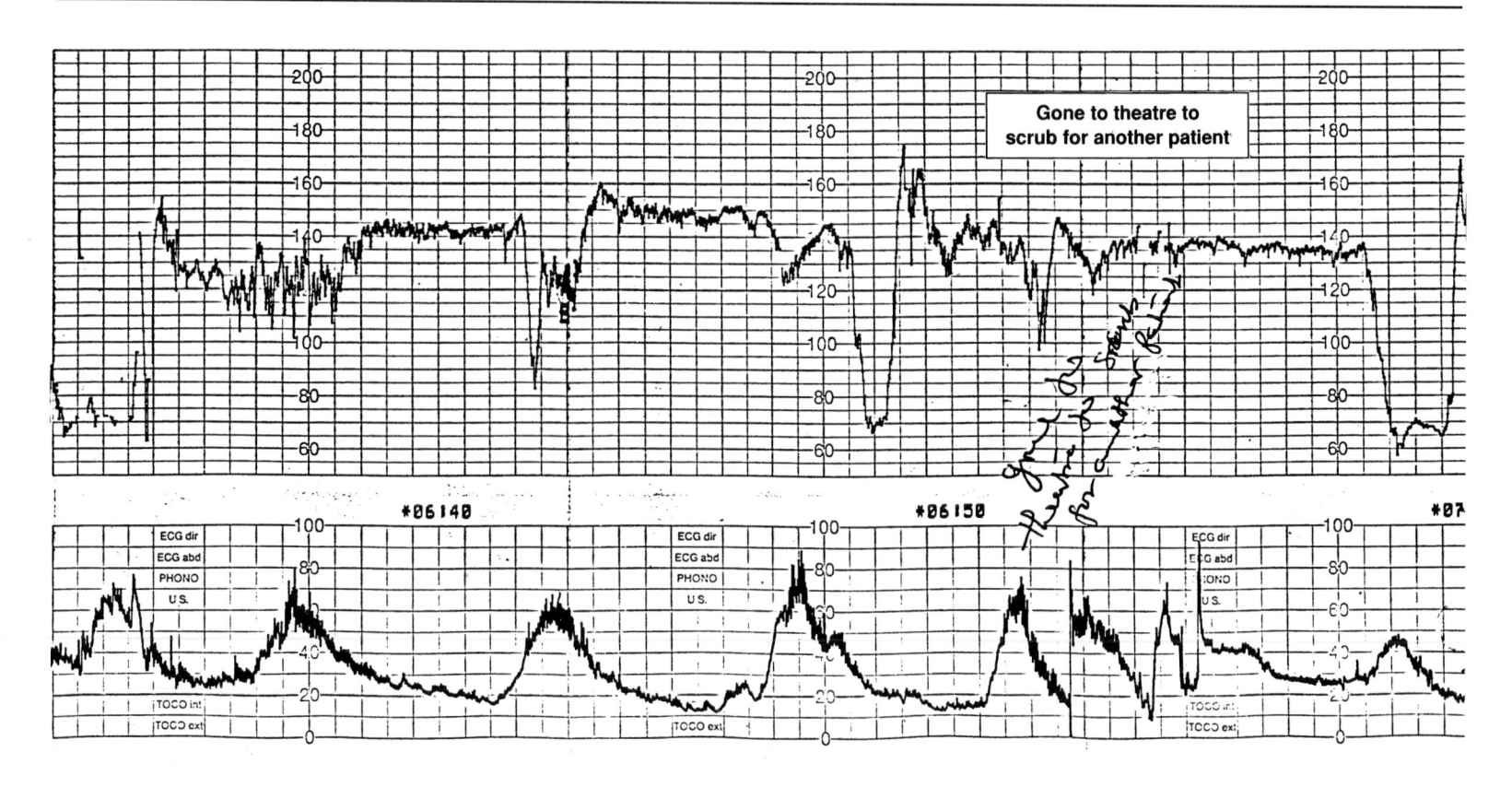

Gone to theatre to
scrub for another patient

*See page 131 for outcome*

08:00    Emergency caesarean section
ROP, no cord entanglement
2.8 kg female
Apgars 9/1 10/5
Right pedunculated fibroid,
outside pelvis

No partogram was kept.

**17.1**
Baseline 140–150 bpm; good variability.
Variable decelerations, mostly Type 1,
broad and deep (dropping 80 bpm) with
accelerations after, suggesting an essentially
healthy fetus but head compression, and
possibly cephalopelvic disproportion
(CPD).

**17.2**
This pattern continues and CPD is
confirmed, resulting in an emergency
caesarean section. Note that the baby only
weighed 2.8 kg but the pelvis felt small and
the position was ROP.

This labour bears certain similarities to
Case 4, and again fetal blood sampling may
have been helpful. However, in contrast to
Case 4, this woman was having good
contractions over several hours, and these
were initially associated with cervical

dilatation to 6 cm. There was then a
secondary arrest of labour and broad,
variable decelerations, with reduced
variability within them, superimposed on
an otherwise reactive trace. This picture is
more in keeping with true CPD, rather
than CPD relative to a malposition of the
fetal head, which may then correct once
adequate contractions are achieved with
oxytocin.

In a primigravid patient, uterine rupture is
rare and so a trial of oxytocin is appropriate,
providing the fetal condition is satisfactory.
If there are worries about CPD one should
reassess cervical progress after 1–2 hours,
and no longer. One must ensure adequate
analgesia before augmenting labour and, if
an operative delivery is thought to be a
possibility, this is an appropriate time to
consider an epidural.

# Clinical points

## AMNIOTOMY

An amniotomy must be performed prior to augmentation of labour, as this reduces the risk of amniotic fluid embolism. Amniotomy also allows visualization of the liquor and hence the presence of meconium. Amniotomy is also often performed prior to the siting of an epidural as it is advisable to apply a fetal scalp electrode when an epidural is sited, as continuous fetal monitoring is essential and the siting of an epidural requires changes in maternal position that may cause loss of contact if an external transducer is employed. Amniotomy is also thought to permit more efficient uterine contractions and improve the rate of cervical dilatation.

## CONTRACTION MONITORING

The external contraction monitor is sensitive to movement, and so, in addition to uterine activity, will pick up voluntary contractions of the abdominal muscles and also the mother changing position. The recording on the CTG indicates the frequency and duration of the contractions, but gives a poor measure of their strength. In order to assess contraction strength accurately it is necessary to use an internal pressure transducer, which is passed into the uterus, alongside the fetal head and away from the placental site. This equipment is not available on all labour wards. It is particularly useful to measure contraction strength when augmenting multiparous patients and in the presence of a uterine scar.

*Cross references:* **Emergency caesarean section** *page 175* **Indications for an epidural** *page 40* **Intrauterine pressure catheter** *page 186*

# CASE 18

35-year Polish, married secretary

G4 P0 +3 (first-trimester TOPs)

EDD 2.6.90

Twin pregnancy
Booked at 13 weeks

Several admissions with raised blood pressure
Good growth on scans
Eventually developed increasing proteinuria

19.5.90 38 weeks

08:00   Labour induced with prostaglandin $E_2$
        Both fetuses cephalic

23:30   Now contracting
        Cervix 1 cm dilated
        Amniotomy performed, clear liquor
        Epidural inserted

04:30   4–5 cm

08:45   7 cm

10:45   8 cm
        Twin 1 right occipito-posterior
        Oxytocin started

13:45   Fully dilated
        Direct occipito-posterior

# 18.1

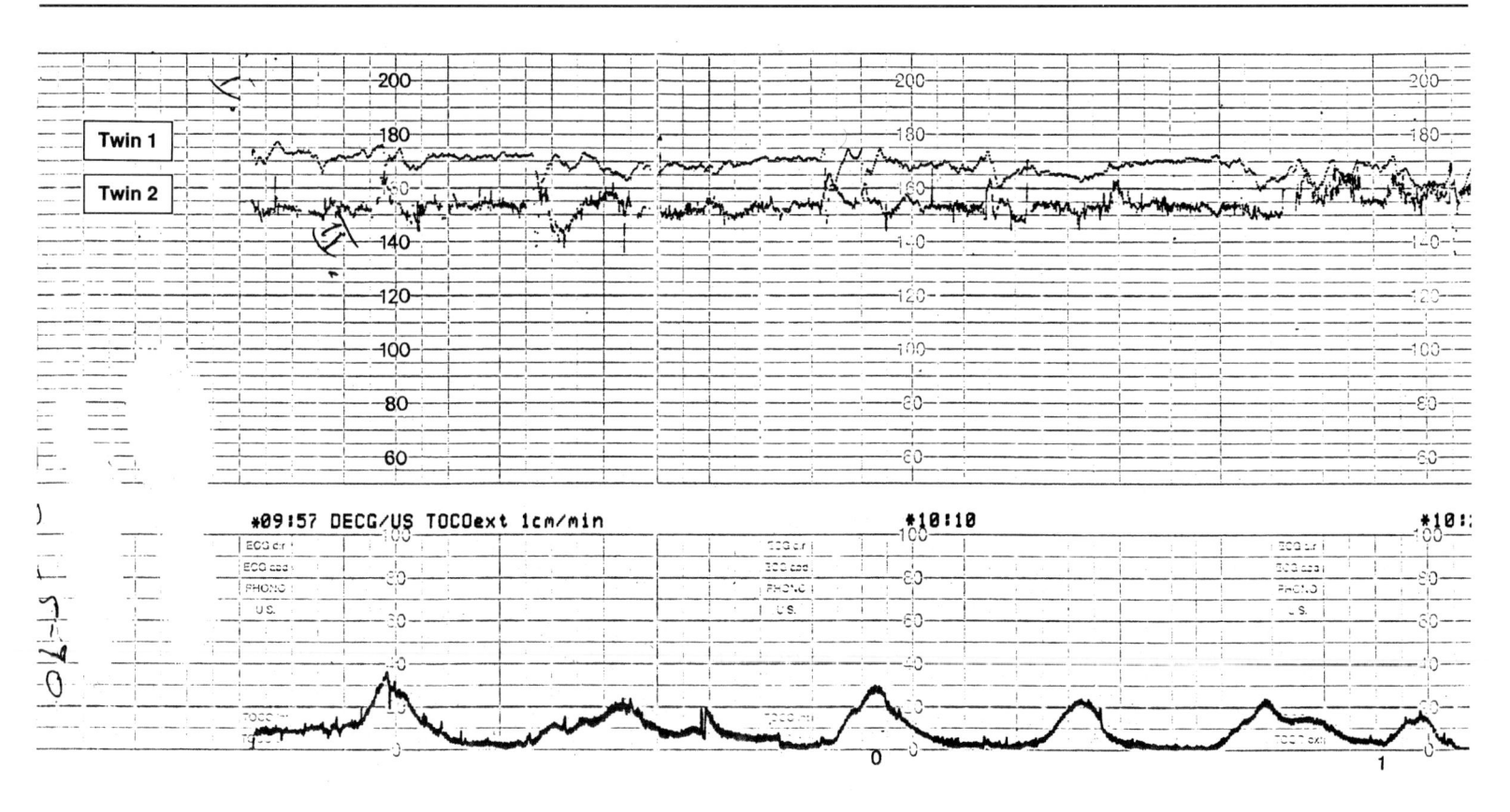

Twin 1

Twin 2

*09:57 DECG/US TOCOext 1cm/min    *10:10    *10:1

ECG cr
ECG abd
PHONO
U.S.

TOCO in

See page 140 for outcome

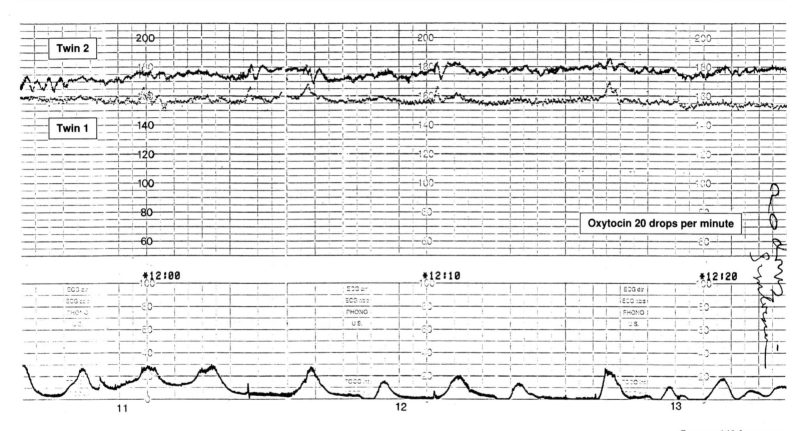

Twin 2

Twin 1

Oxytocin 20 drops per minute

*12:00    *12:10    *12:20

11    12    13

*See page 140 for outcome*

# 18.3

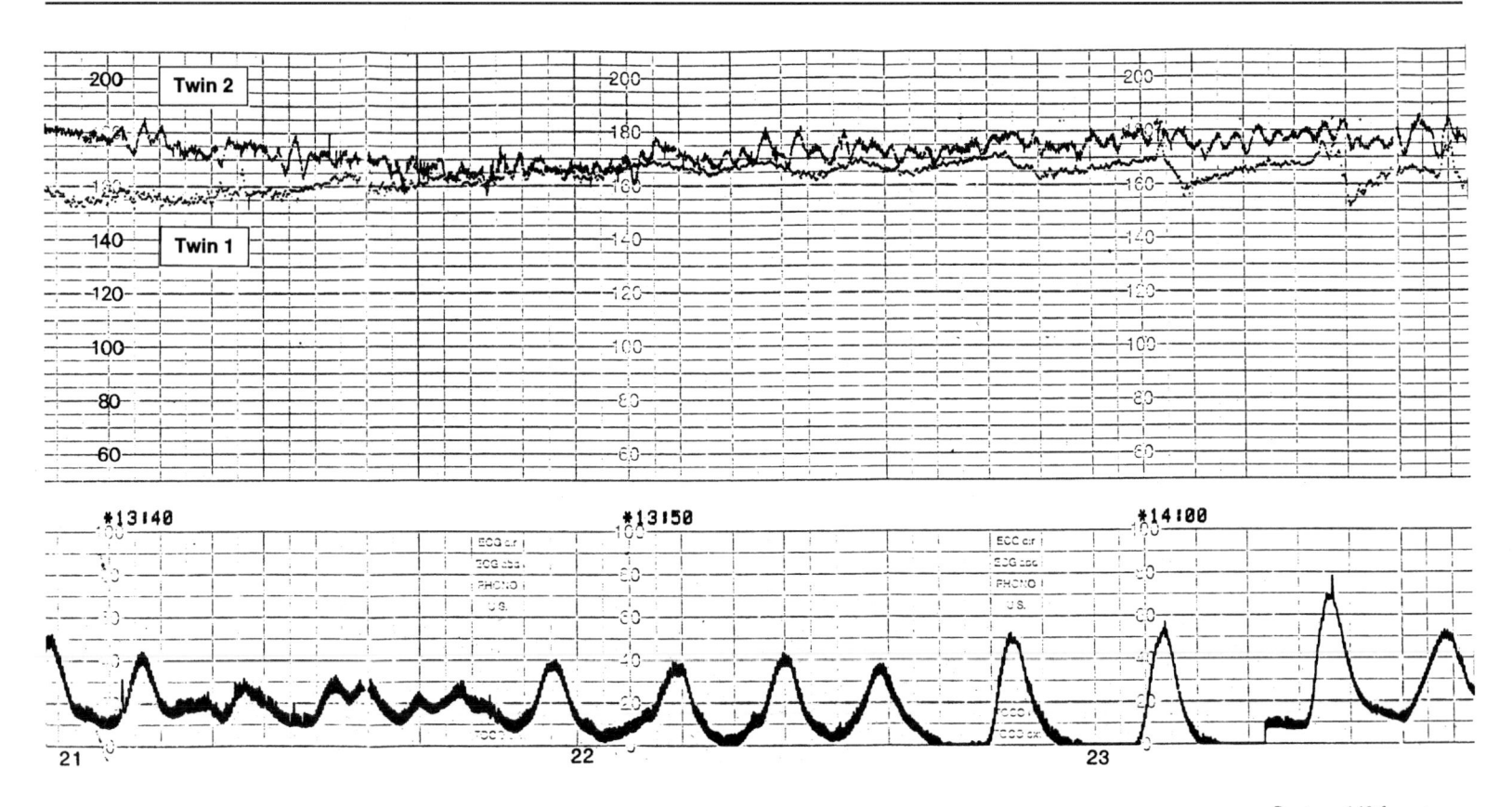

*See page 140 for outcome*

# 18.4

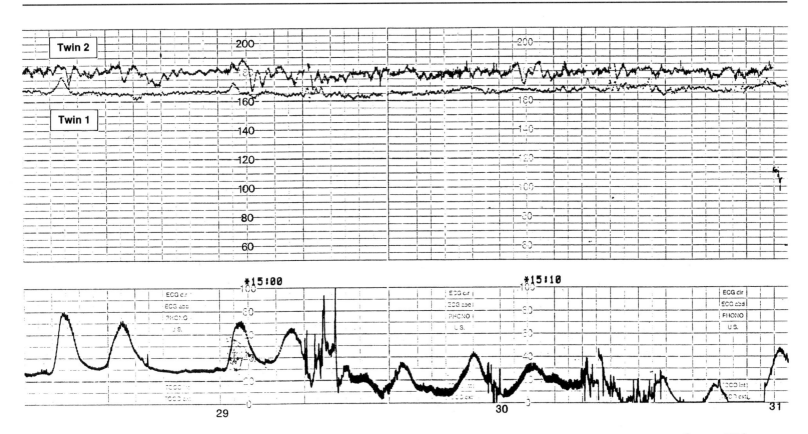

*See page 140 for outcome*

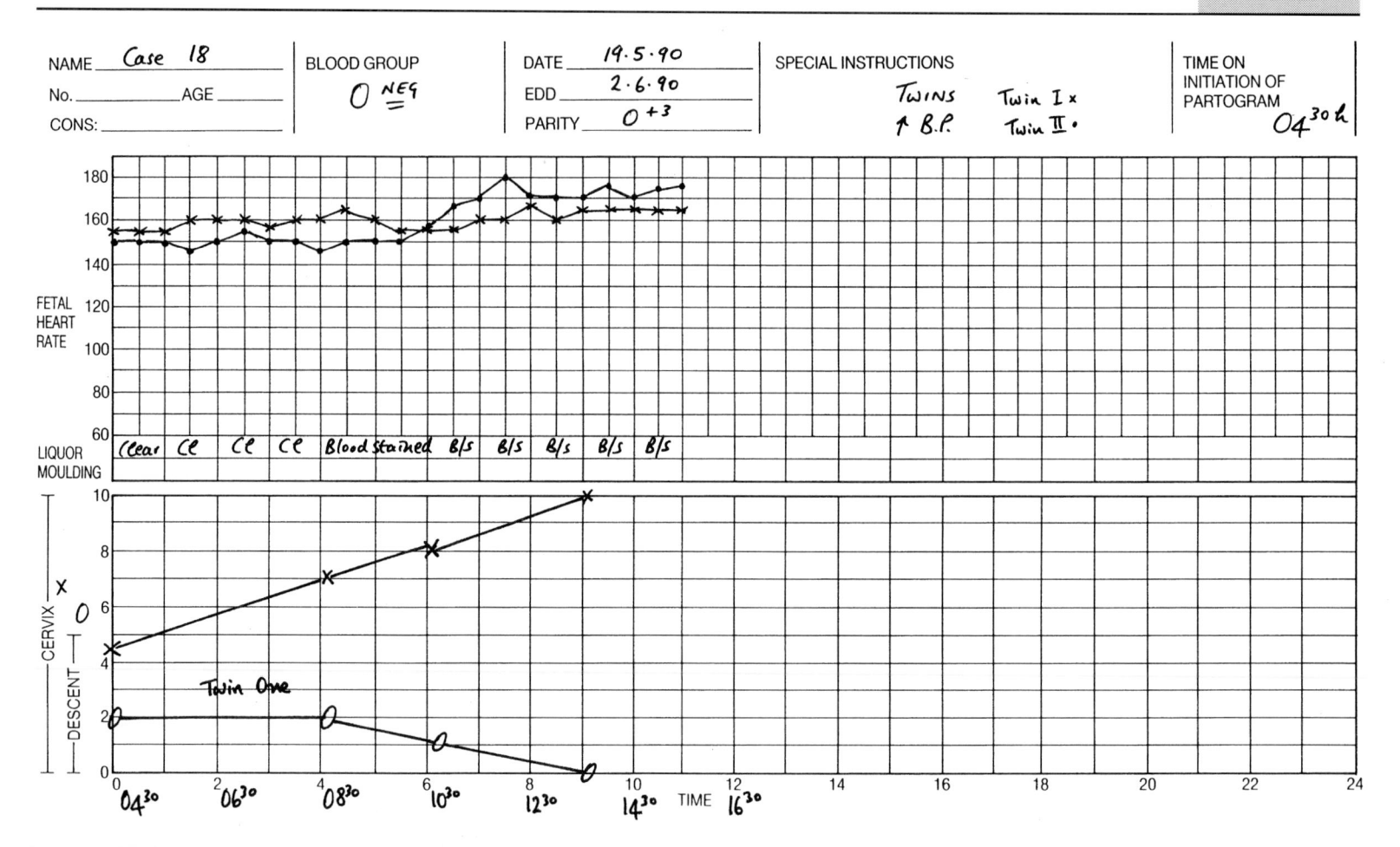

NAME _Case 18_

No. _____ AGE _____

CONS: _____

BLOOD GROUP

$O \underset{=}{NEG}$

DATE _19.5.90_

EDD _2.6.90_

PARITY _O +3_

SPECIAL INSTRUCTIONS

_TWINS_   _Twin I x_

↑ _B.P._   _Twin II •_

TIME ON INITIATION OF PARTOGRAM

_04³⁰ h_

**FETAL HEART RATE**

180 — 160 — 140 — 120 — 100 — 80 — 60

**LIQUOR MOULDING**

| Clear | Cl | Cl | Cl | Blood stained | B/s | B/s | B/s | B/s | B/s |

**CERVIX** x

**O**

**DESCENT**

Twin One

TIME

04³⁰   06³⁰   08³⁰   10³⁰   12³⁰   14³⁰   16³⁰

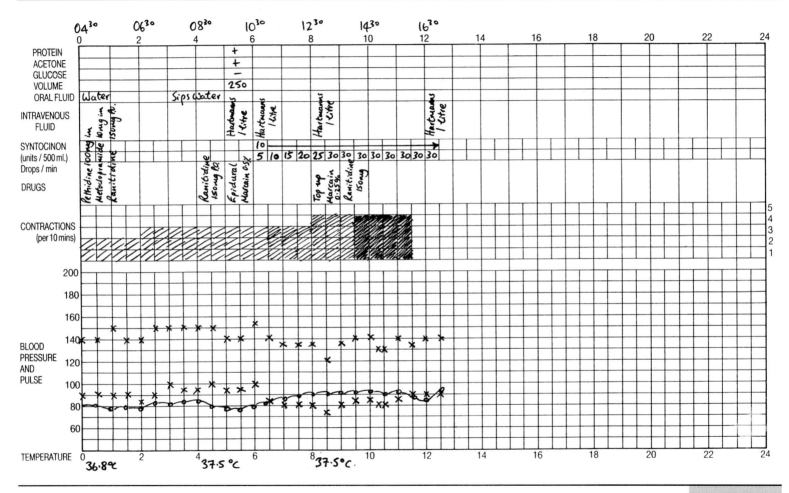

# Outcome

15:35   Ventouse delivery twin 1
        2.95 kg male
        Apgars 7/1 9/5  10/10

15:46   Neville–Barnes forceps delivery
        twin 2
        2.42 kg male
        Apgars 5/1 6/5 8/10 10/20

The partogram appears to have been
started 4 hours too late.

**18.1**
Twin 1—baseline 170 bpm
    2—baseline 150 bpm

Both show occasional shallow decelerations
and reduced variability, but this may be an
artefact of the twin monitor which tends to
damp down the sensitivity of the recording.

**18.2**
Twin 2 is now faster than twin 1.

**18.3**
Twin 2 has better variability, twin 1 is
beginning to show shallow Type 2
decelerations.

**18.4**
Both fetuses appear to be stable and coping
well with labour just before delivery.

# Clinical points

## MONITORING LABOUR IN MULTIPLE PREGNANCY

In a twin labour it is very important to be able to monitor both fetuses simultaneously. Two external transducers often interfere with each other electronically, so the best solution is to put a fetal scalp electrode on twin 1 (dots) and an external transducer on twin 2 and use a special twin monitor, as in this case. This way one can also see both traces at the same time and be certain that each fetus is being monitored.

Monitoring twins prior to membrane rupture is best achieved after first localizing the position of each heart by ultrasound. Before the onset of labour a biophysical profile is a good way to assess the other physiological variables in each fetus without having the difficulty of relying solely upon obtaining simultaneous CTG traces.

## TERMINATING THE CTG RECORDING

It is a good idea not to tear the paper from the CTG machine the moment that the baby delivers, as a few minutes of blank recording shows that the trace has not been ended prematurely to hide a second stage abnormality. This may be important if medicolegal problems arise.

## TRIPLETS AND MORE

One of the reasons for usually performing a caesarean section for triplets, and higher order multiple pregnancies, is the difficulty in monitoring them during labour.

## MATERNAL SIZE AND TRANSDUCER MOVEMENT

When an external transducer is being used, a sudden drop in the fetal heart rate may indicate loss of contact with the transmitted pulse rather than a bradycardia. This is particularly likely in overweight women, or women with multiple pregnancies, in whom movement easily results in slippage of the transducer so that the pulse in the maternal aorta is detected instead of the fetal heart.

*Cross references:* **Epidurals** *pages 33, 40, 90* **The biophysical profile** *page 86*

# CASE 19

| | |
|---|---|
| 20-year single, unemployed | **12.6.90** 41+ weeks |
| Primigravida | **18:05** Admitted with irregular contractions<br>Cephalic presentation<br>Left occipito-anterior (LOA) position<br>Head 1/5 palpable<br>Cervix (Cx) thick, long and closed |
| EDD 1.6.90 | |
| Booked 12 weeks | |
| Uneventful pregnancy | **13.6.90** |
| | **01:30** Cx 3–4 cm dilated, membranes bulging |
| | **02:30** 4 cm, amniotomy, clear liquor<br>Fetal scalp electrode applied<br>Epidural |
| | **08:45** 5 cm dilated<br>LOA position<br>Oxytocin started |
| | **10:50** Fully dilated |

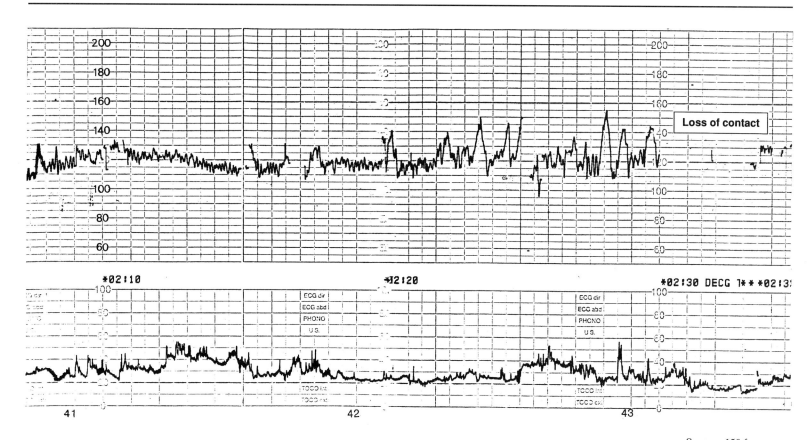

Loss of contact

*See page 150 for outcome*

# 19.2

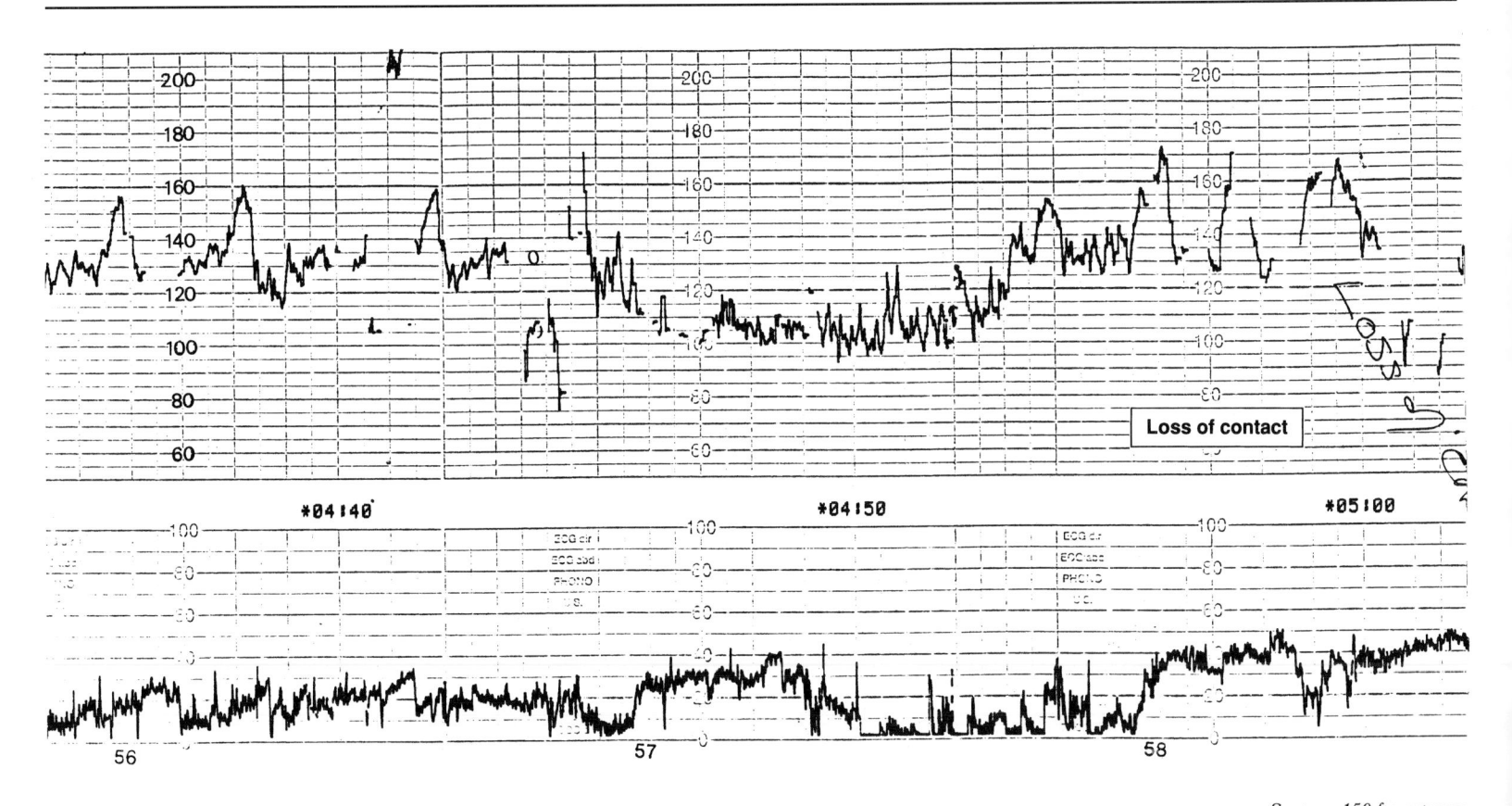

**Loss of contact**

*See page 150 for outcome*

# 19.3

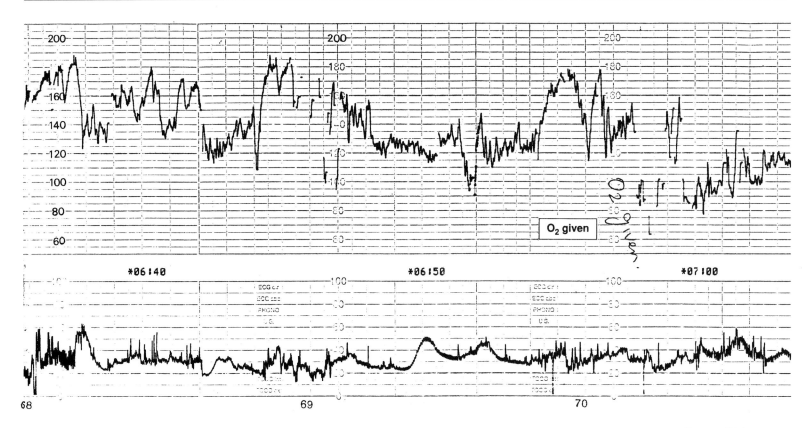

*O₂ given*

O₂ given

*See page 150 for outcome*

## 19.4

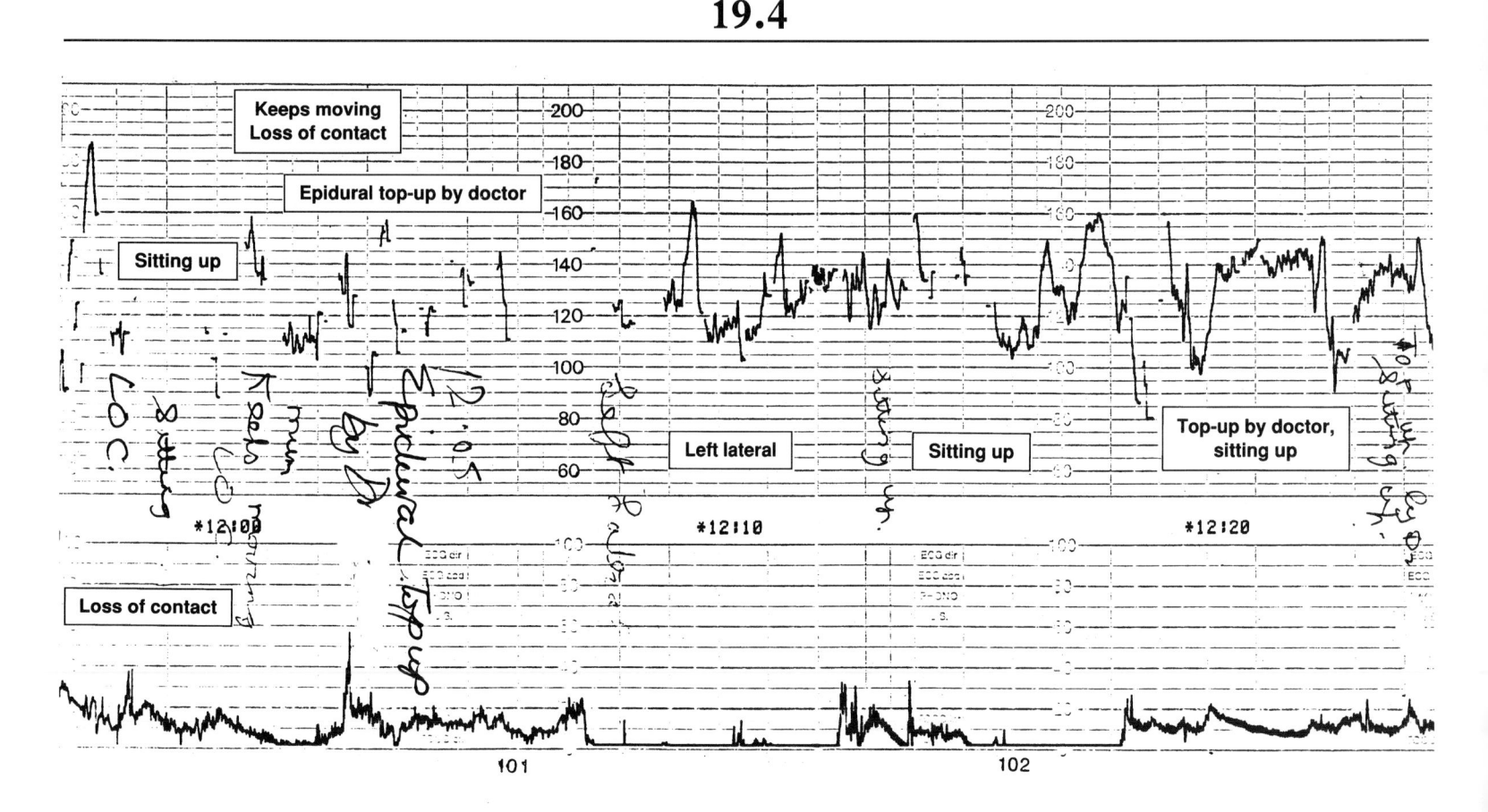

*See page 150 for outcome*

# 19.5

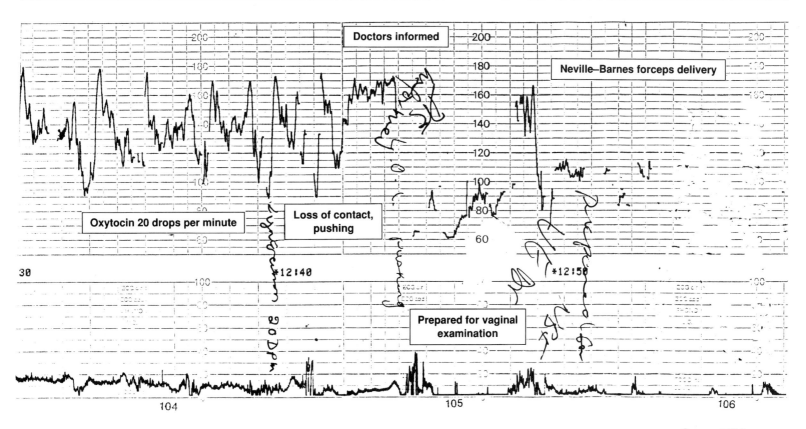

**Doctors informed**

**Neville–Barnes forceps delivery**

**Oxytocin 20 drops per minute**

**Loss of contact, pushing**

**Prepared for vaginal examination**

*See page 150 for outcome*

**CASE 19**

NAME _Case 19_
No. _____ AGE _20y_
CONS: _____

BLOOD GROUP
_A Pos_

DATE _13.6.90_
EDD _1.6.90_
PARITY _0 +o_

SPECIAL INSTRUCTIONS

TIME ON
INITIATION OF
PARTOGRAM
_02³⁰ ᵘ_

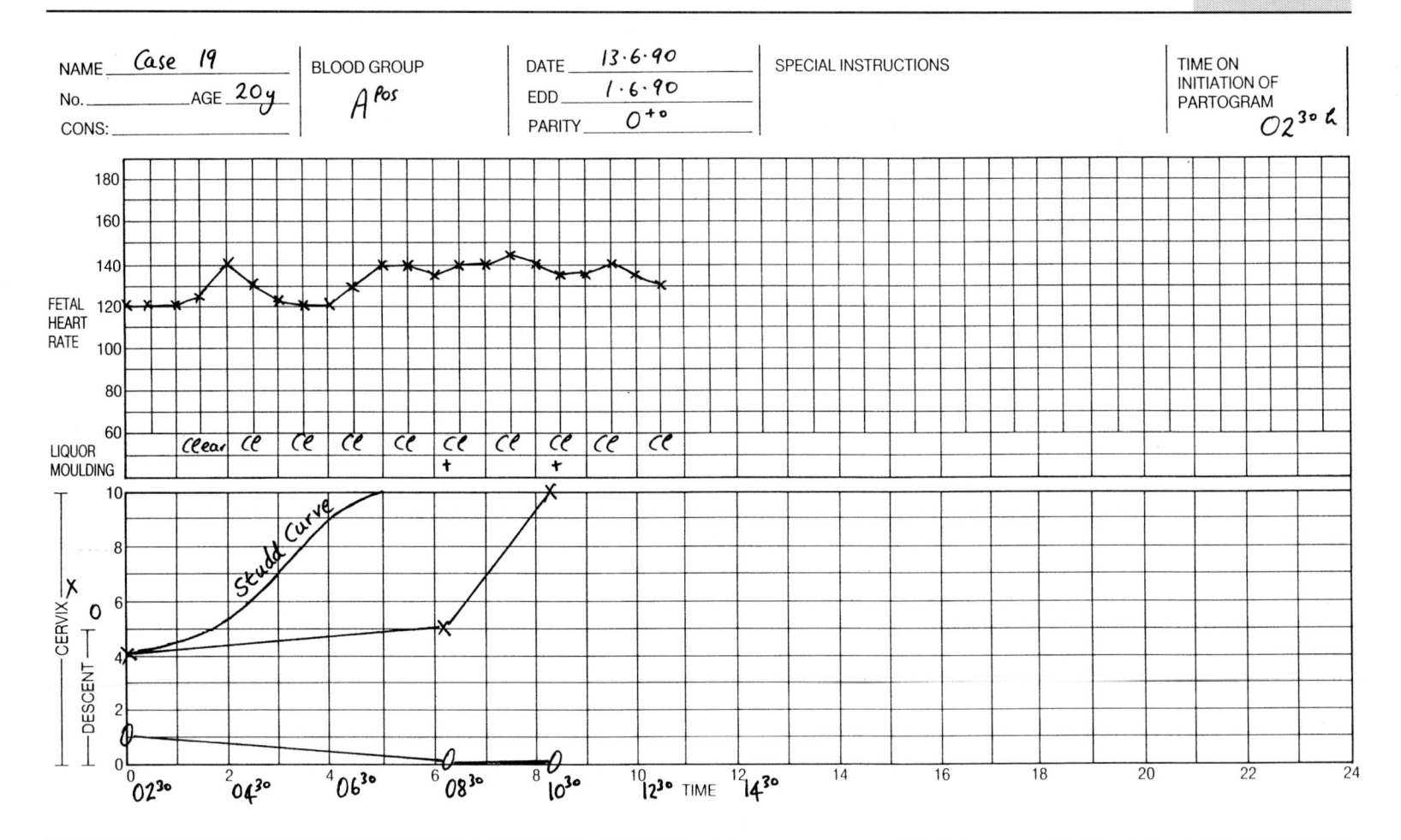

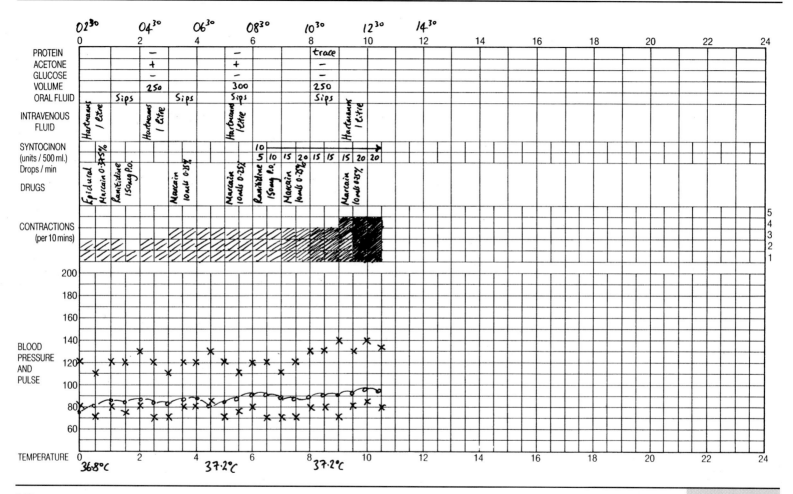

CASE 19

# Outcome

12:50   Neville–Barnes forceps delivery
        3.87 kg male
        Apgars 8/1 10/5

This is another case of primary dysfunctional labour in a primigravida, which responded to oxytocin and required a forceps delivery for a prolonged second stage.

**19.1**
Rate 120 bpm, good variability with accelerations.

**19.2**
Superimposed on a reactive trace there is a bradycardia of 110 bpm, still with good variability.

**19.3**
There is good reactivity, large accelerations and a further bradycardia.

**19.4**
Such loss of contact should not occur with an epidural if there is a fetal scalp electrode.

**19.5**
After a further prolonged bradycardia a simple forceps delivery was performed.

# Clinical points

## THE FETAL SCALP ELECTRODE

The two commonly used types of fetal scalp electrode (FSE) are the spiral double helix and the Copeland clip. Both pick up the fetal electrocardiogram (ECG), but rather than record the entire ECG waveform the machinery is designed to record the R wave only, so that a heart rate is printed, in the same way as with the external transducer.

The advantage of an FSE is that the fetus may be monitored continuously without the loss of contact and discomfort that may occur with the external transducer. It is applied during a vaginal examination and should not cause the mother discomfort. That it hurts the baby is shown by a brief acceleration in heart rate after it has been applied (used by some as a sign of fetal responsiveness and well-being), yet this appears to be short-lived, and we assume that the fetal scalp is used to intense pressure during labour and delivery, so that

the small clip should not cause prolonged pain. It is important to avoid placing the FSE directly over a fontanelle, as here there is no bone beneath the skin and hence a potential risk of introducing infection. The FSE very rarely causes long-term problems to the baby and has not been found to introduce infection to the mother. It has been suggested that the FSE should be avoided in pregnancies that are high risk for human immunodeficiency virus infection, as there is a potential risk of transmission from the mother to the fetus.

If telemetry is available it is possible for the mother to remain mobile whilst an FSE is being used (see page 1).

Always remember to remove the FSE prior to an instrumental delivery, and *especially* before a caesarean section (when monitoring should be continued with an external transducer until the operation starts).

## OTHER METHODS OF CONTINUOUS MONITORING

In recent years much research has been directed towards more reliable means of continuous fetal monitoring that provide a better indication of fetal health than the simple change in heart rate recorded by the CTG. Details of these methods, which are still being evaluated, are beyond the scope of this book, they include:
—Fetal electrocardiogram
—Fetal electroencephalogram
—Continuous biochemical monitoring
—Pulse oximetry

*Cross references:*   **Epidurals** *pages 33, 40, 99*   **Continuous monitoring** *page 90*

# CASE 20

31-year Jamaican housewife

G8 P5 +2

| | |
|---|---|
| 1976 | NVD 3.40 kg female |
| 1977 | NVD 3.57 kg female |
| 1980 | NVD 3.57 kg male |
| 1982 | Termination of pregnancy |
| 1983 | NVD 3.66 kg female |
| 1986 | Termination of pregnancy |
| 1988 | NVD 3.15 kg male |

No other history

EDD 25.4.90 by scan

Booked at 15 weeks

29.4.90 40+ weeks

| | |
|---|---|
| 17:00 | Admitted, thought to be in early labour<br>Head high, 4/5 palpable<br>Cervix long and closed |
| 22:10 | No change in cervix, contractions stronger |
| 24:10 | Still no change |

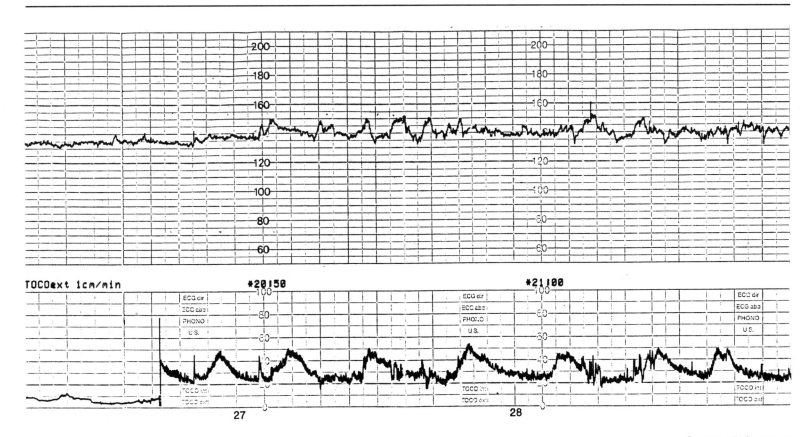

TOCOext 1cm/min

#20150　　　　　　　#21100

ECG dir
ECG abd
PHONO
U.S.

TOCO int
TOCO ext

27　　　　　　28

*See page 156 for outcome*

## 20.2

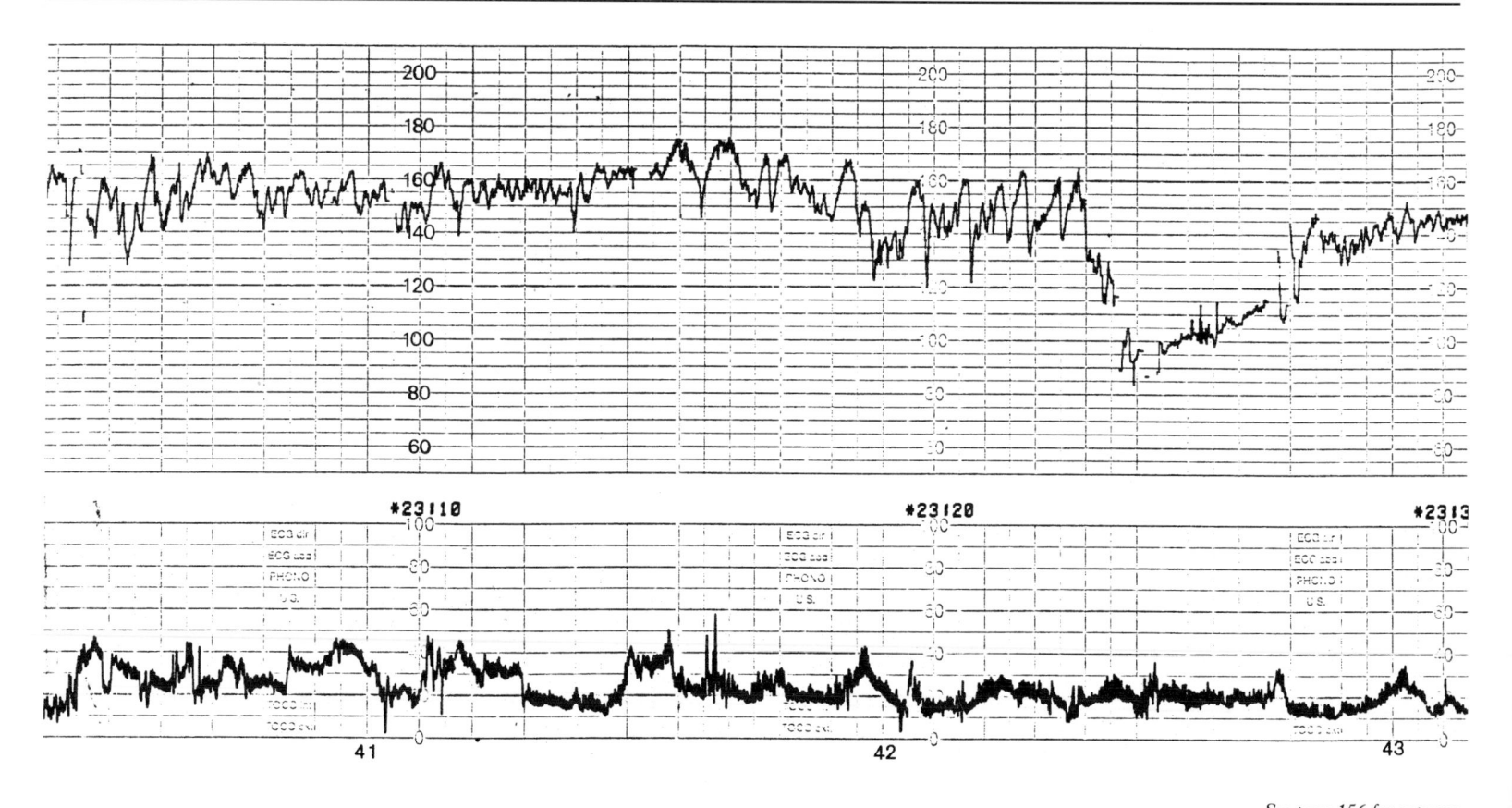

*See page 156 for outcome*

# 20.3

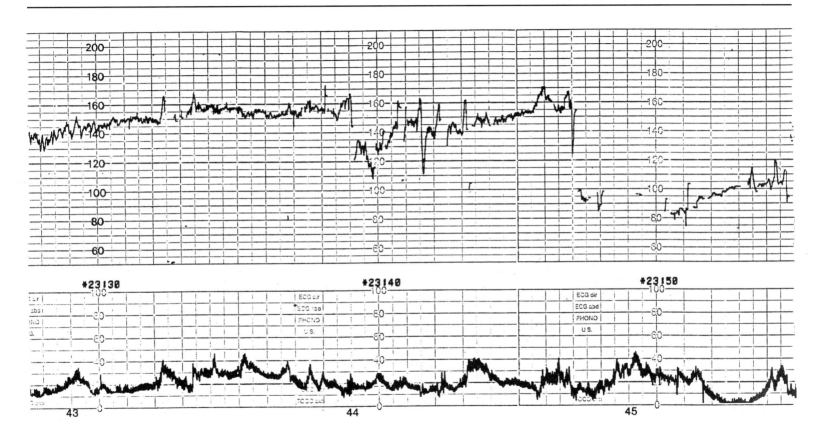

*See page 156 for outcome*

**CASE 20**

# Outcome

00:30 Emergency caesarean section
3.94 kg female
Apgars 6/1 9/5
Fresh meconium, cord once
around neck

No partogram was kept.

Grand multiparas often present with
unexpected problems. This infant was
quite a bit larger than her previous babies.

**20.1**
Baseline 135–140 bpm, reactive trace.

**20.2**
Baseline 150–160 bpm; swings in the heart
rate greater than 25 bpm are said to be
'saltatory' and indicate loss of control over
the fetal cardiovascular system. There is
a period of bradycardia to 100 bpm for
4 minutes. On balance we would not be
too worried about this trace.

**20.3**
There is initially reduced variability with
small accelerations; then there is a further
bradycardia.

In spite of apparently adequate
contractions, there was no cervical progress
and there were signs of fetal distress. The
head was not engaged and caesarean
section was obviously the right decision.

# Clinical points

## GRAND MULTIPARITY

Women in their fifth pregnancy, or greater, have an increased incidence of maternal and perinatal mortality. The older women is also more likely to be anaemic, have hypertension and develop gestational diabetes. Placenta praevia and multiple pregnancies are more common, and the multiparous, hypotonic uterus may result in a malpresentation or an unstable lie, with the risks of cord prolapse and operative delivery. Progressively larger babies increase the risk of obstructed labour and uterine rupture, and postpartum haemorrhage is also more likely.

## TUBAL LIGATION

Tubal ligation was offered to this woman, but declined. One should always balance the benefits of sterilization at the time of a caesarean section, namely the avoidance of further anaesthesia and the possibility of difficulties with laparoscopy in a pelvis that has been operated on, with the increased failure rate associated with the vascular fallopian tubes of pregnancy and, more importantly, uncertainty about the infant's condition, especially at an emergency operation.

It is worthwhile discussing this issue in the antenatal clinic, in anticipation of a possible caesarean section. This allows time for the mother to think it over and discuss sterilization with her partner, rather than be confronted with having to make a rushed decision on the labour ward.

Cross references:    **Meconium**  pages 33, 48    **Saltatory heart rate**  page 3

**CASE 20**

# CASE 21

22-year single, secretary

G3 P0 +2 (TOPs)

No other history

EDD 30.5.90 by scan

Booked 14 weeks

Uneventful pregnancy

---

30.5.90 40 weeks

Admitted thought to be contracting
Cervix (Cx) undilated
Later allowed to go home,
as not in labour

3.6.90   Readmitted with a 'show'
Cephalic presentation
Left occipito-anterior (LOA)
position
Head 2/5 palpable

09:00   Cx 2 cm dilated, mild contractions

---

4.6.90   Contractions settled, but decision
to induce as postdates

14:30   3 cm

16:25   5 cm
Amniotomy, clear liquor
Left occipito-transverse (LOT)
Epidural

18:25   Ephedrine given for drop in
blood pressure

19:30   7 cm
LOT

22:50   Head 0/5 palpable
9+ cm
LOA

23:30   Prolonged decelerations

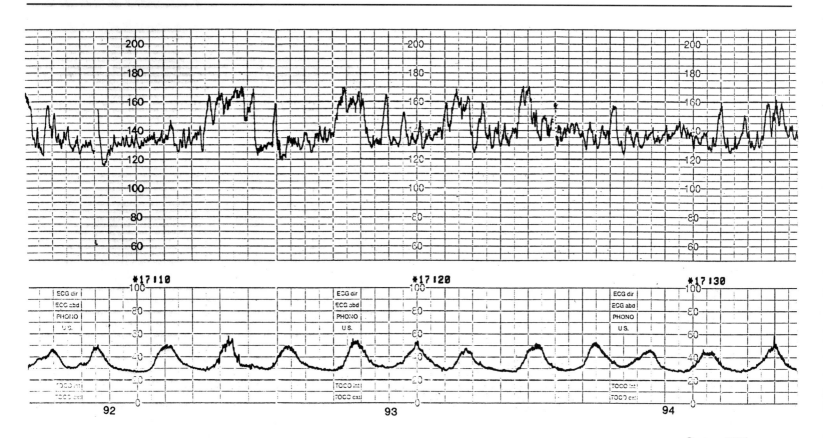

*See page 166 for outcome*

# 21.2

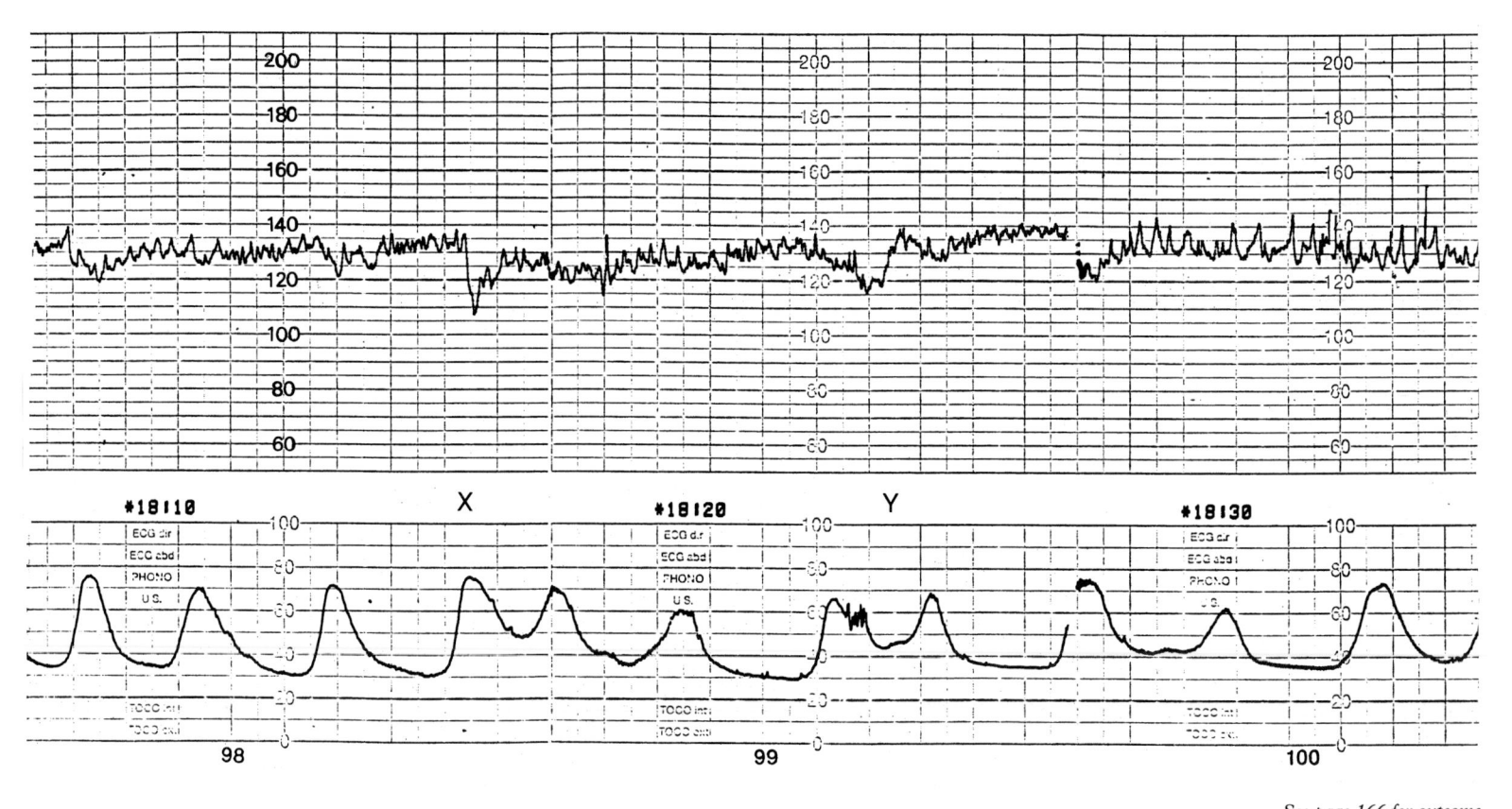

*See page 166 for outcome*

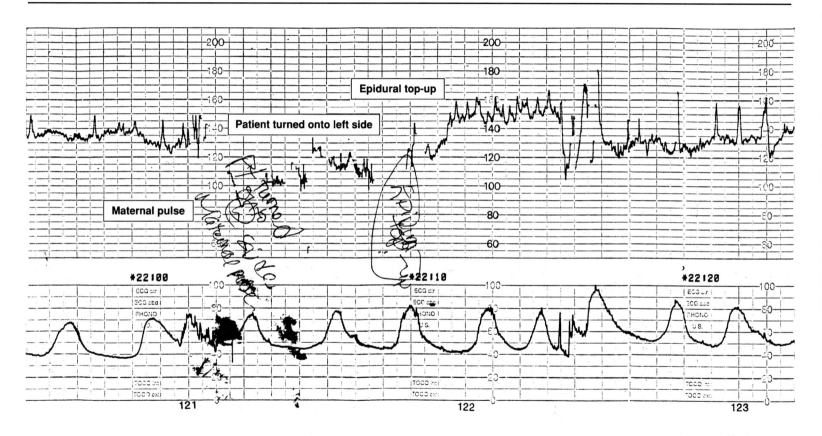

Epidural top-up

Patient turned onto left side

Maternal pulse

*See page 166 for outcome*

# 21.4

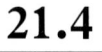

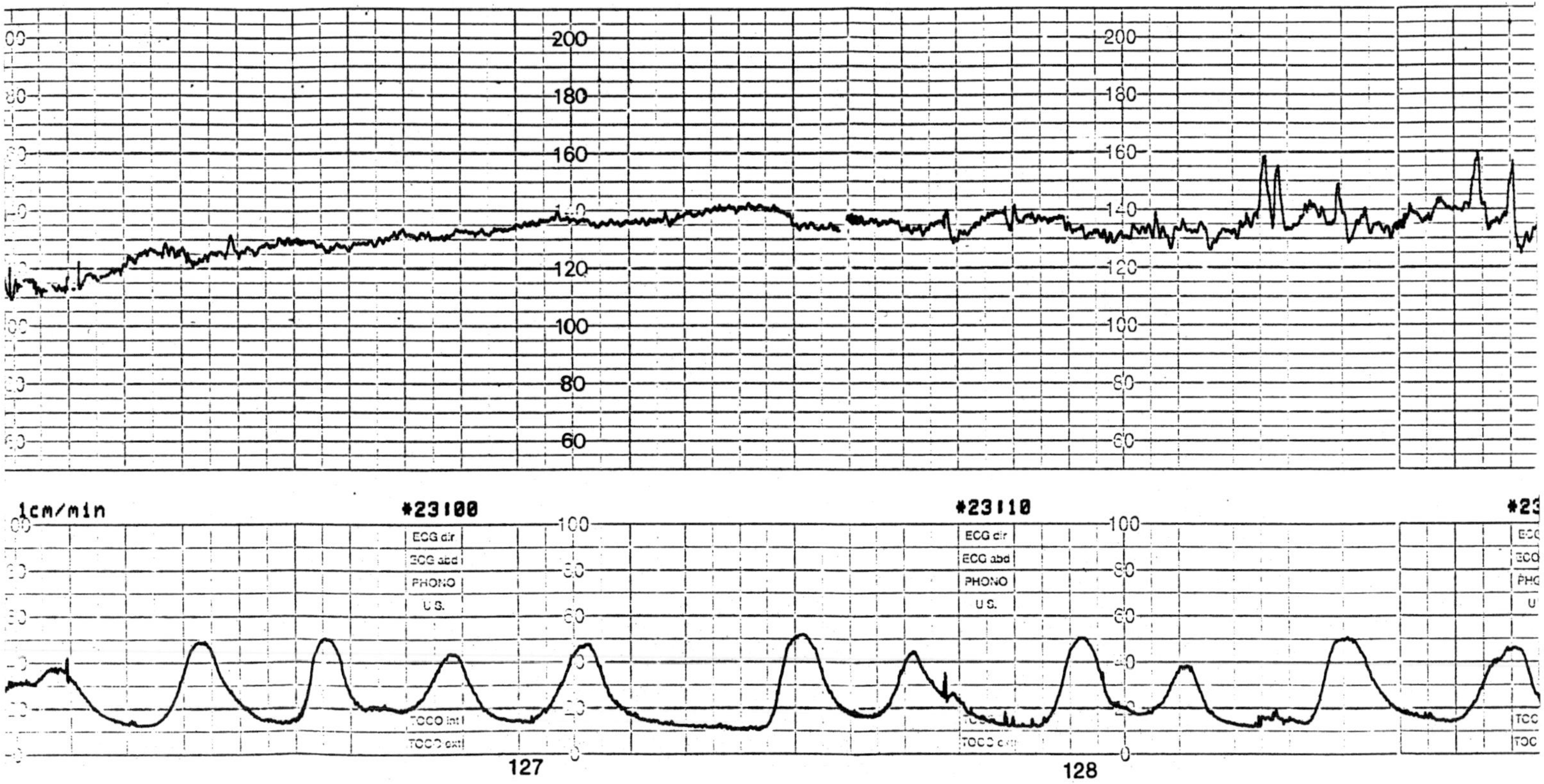

1cm/min

#23100

#23110

#23

127

128

*See page 166 for outcome*

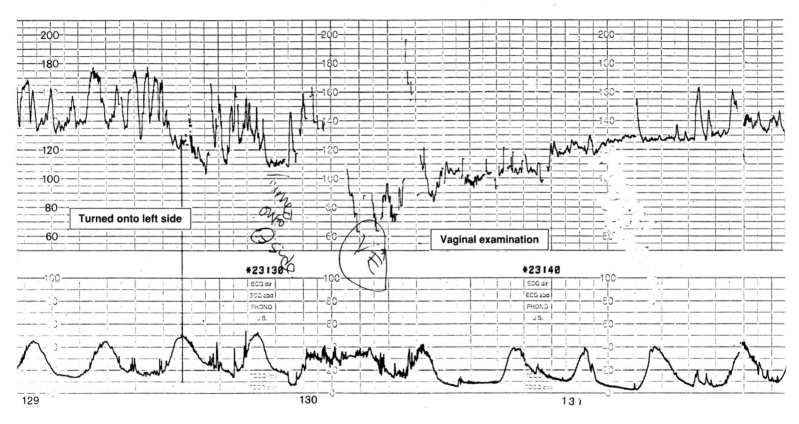

Turned onto left side

Vaginal examination

#23130

#23140

*See page 166 for outcome*

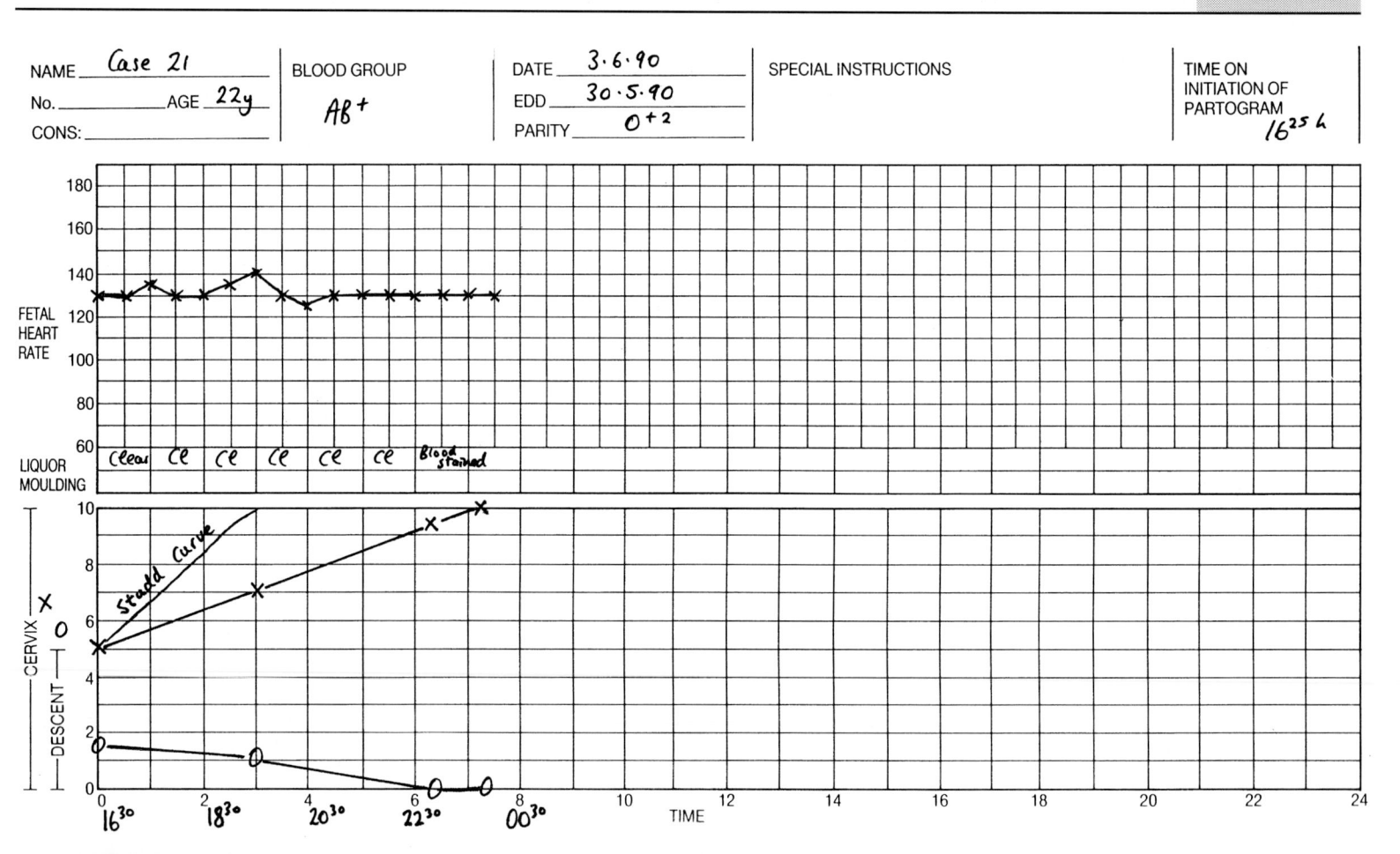

NAME _Case 21_

No. _____ AGE _22y_

CONS: _____

BLOOD GROUP

_AB +_

DATE _3.6.90_

EDD _30.5.90_

PARITY _0 +2_

SPECIAL INSTRUCTIONS

TIME ON
INITIATION OF
PARTOGRAM

_16²⁵ h_

FETAL HEART RATE

LIQUOR MOULDING: Clear | Cℓ | Cℓ | Cℓ | Cℓ | Cℓ | Blood stained

CERVIX / DESCENT

Stadd Curve

TIME

16³⁰  18³⁰  20³⁰  22³⁰  00³⁰

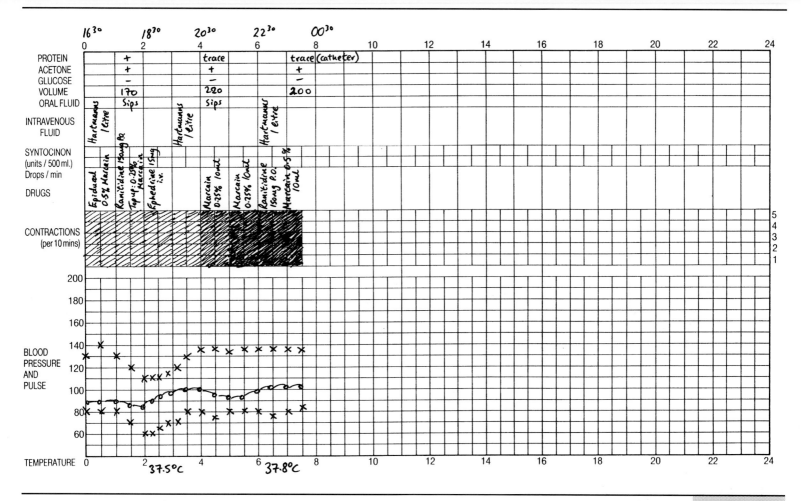

# Outcome

23:45   Ventouse delivery
        4.21 kg male
        Apgars good
        No cord entanglement

The partogram was started too late.

Note the large size of the baby.

**21.1**
Baseline 130 bpm, very reactive with accelerations.

**21.2**
Baseline 130, reactive; X is a Type 1 and Y a Type 2 deceleration, but the trace at this stage suggests a healthy fetus.

**21.3**
This period of bradycardia may be related to head rotation (LOT at 7 cm, LOA at 9 cm).

**21.4**
After a deceleration (just finishing), variability is suddenly reduced—this could represent either rest–activity cycling or fetal distress. Uterine activity is less regular, suggesting relative cephalopelvic disproportion.

**21.5**
This is a saltatory trace followed by a further bradycardia. In view of the full dilatation it was decided to proceed to ventouse delivery. It is debatable as to whether this was performed prematurely as the trace does not indicate severe fetal compromise.

# Clinical points

## APGAR SCORES

The Apgar score provides an immediate assessment of the baby's neonatal condition and is measured 1, 5, 10 and sometimes 20 minutes after delivery. A poor Apgar score indicates the need for resuscitative measures but is unreliable in its prediction of long term outcome.

The Apgar score is calculated as follows:

|  | Score | | |
|---|---|---|---|
|  | 0 | 1 | 2 |
| Heart rate | absent | less than 100 | more than 100 |
| Respirations | absent | weak cry | strong cry |
| Muscle tone | limp | some flexion | active motion |
| Reflex irritability | absent | grimace | cry |
| Colour | blue/pale | pink body, blue peripheries | pink |

## INDICATIONS FOR THE PRESENCE OF A PAEDIATRICIAN AT DELIVERY

1. Preterm baby (less than 37 completed weeks)
2. Intrauterine growth retardation
3. Prolonged rupture of membranes (more than 24 hours)
4. Fetal distress
5. Meconium stained liquor
6. Operative/instrumental delivery (except elective caesarean section for non-fetal reasons)
7. Breech
8. Multiple pregnancy (one paediatrician for each baby)
9. Fetal abnormality (of whatever nature)
10. Maternal illness—chronic, e.g. diabetes mellitus —acute, e.g. antepartum haemorrhage, severe pre-eclampsia

# Clinical points

## RESUSCITATION OF THE NEWBORN

All midwives and doctors should be conversant with basic neonatal resuscitation. When necessary this should be initiated without delay, whilst awaiting the arrival of a paediatrician.

### Apgar score 6–7
—Dry the baby, keep him warm, cover his head
—Clear the mouth and nostrils (too vigorous suction may cause laryngeal spasm)
—Give facial oxygen
—Stimulate the soles of the feet

If breathing is not established and pethidine was administered to mother within the last 6 hours, give naloxone (0.2 mg intramuscularly if over 2.5 kg, 0.1 mg if less than 2.5 kg).
In presence of meconium, aspirate the mouth and nostrils as the head delivers then try to splint the chest after delivery and aspirate below the vocal cords before the first inspiration.

### Apgar score 3–5
—As above, plus intermittent positive-pressure oxygen using a face-mask and bag
—Intubate if the heart rate remains below 100 bpm or if there is no spontaneous breath by 4 minutes

### Apgar score 0–2
—Intubate: 30 respirations/minute; first inflation pressure 30 cm water, then 20 cm water
—If the heart rate does not improve start external massage (100 bpm)
—If still unresponsive give drugs: Adrenaline 1:10 000 (0.1 ml per kg) down endotracheal tube or parenterally Sodium bicarbonate 4.2%, 2 ml/kg, 25% dextrose (if blood sugar is less than 2.5 mmol/l)

# CASE 22

22-year Irish, single

Primigravida
No past history

EDD 17.5.90

Booked late at 26 weeks

Hb 9.3 g/dl at booking rising to
at term
Otherwise, uneventful pregnancy

26.5.90 41+ weeks

Admitted with possible ruptured
membranes—unconfirmed, not
contracting

27.5.90 Discharged

28.5.90 Readmitted contracting

05:30   Cervix 3 cm dilated
          Intact membranes

08:30   5 cm

10:50   7 cm
          Amniotomy, clear liquor
          Pethidine given

14:50   8 cm
          Oxytocin started

16:30   8 cm
          More pethidine given

18:20   8 cm
          Epidural sited
          Position of head undefined

# 22.1

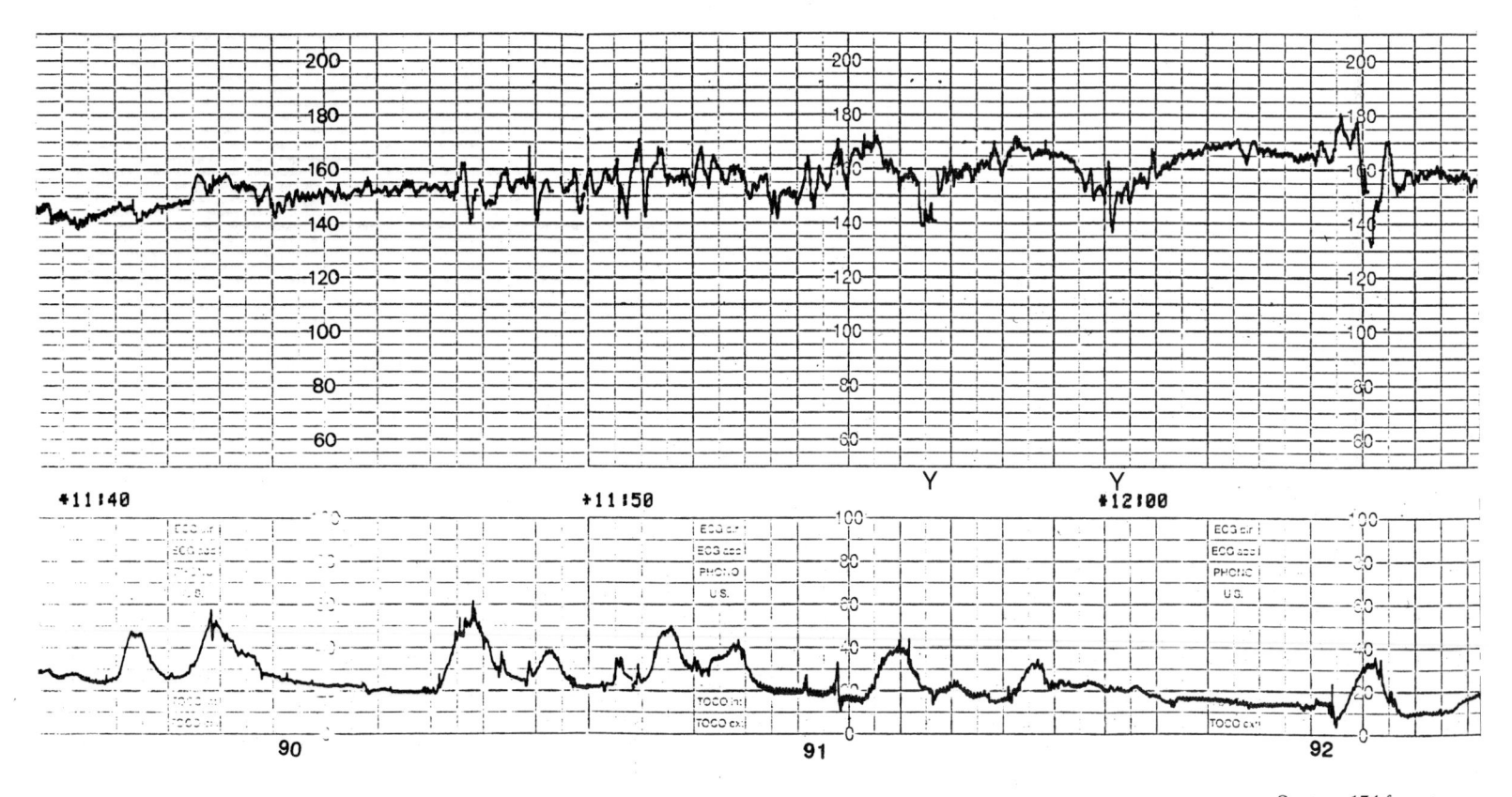

See page 174 for outcome

# 22.2

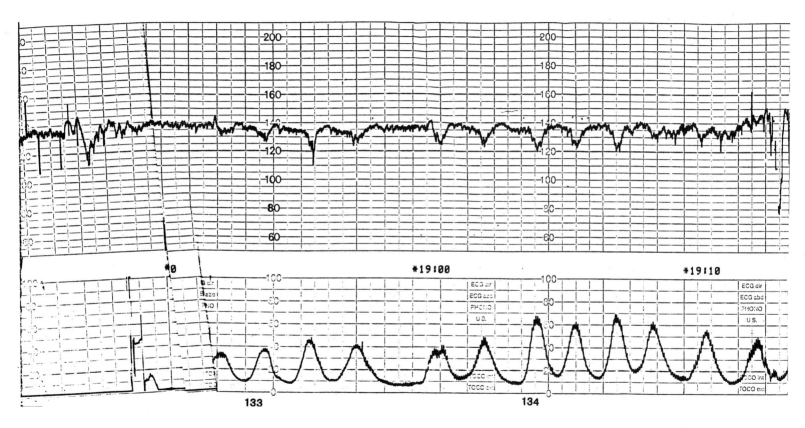

*See page 174 for outcome*

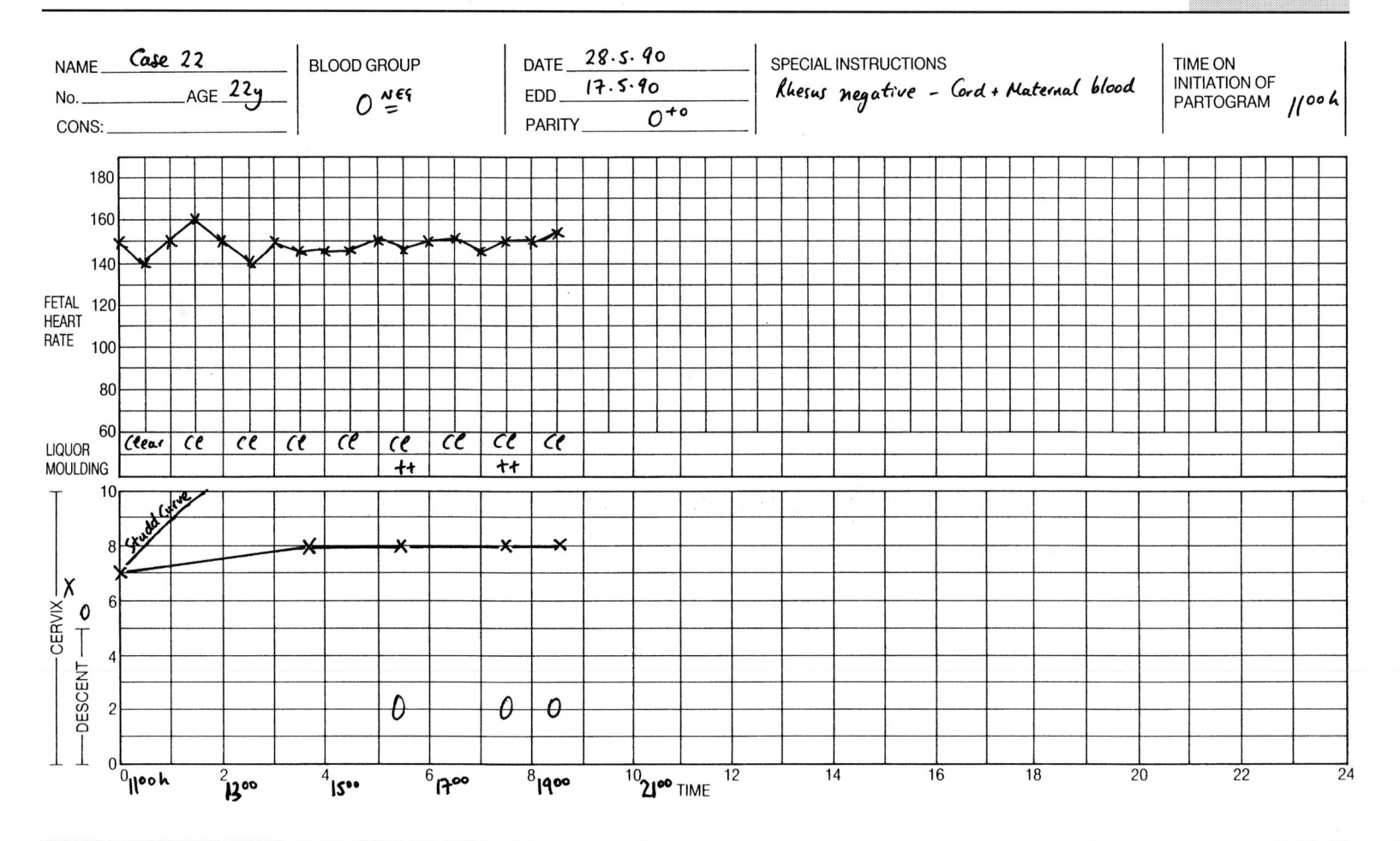

NAME _Case 22_

No. _____ AGE _22y_

CONS: _____

BLOOD GROUP

$O \overset{NEG}{=}$

DATE _28.5.90_

EDD _17.5.90_

PARITY _0⁺⁰_

SPECIAL INSTRUCTIONS

_Rhesus negative - Cord + Maternal blood_

TIME ON INITIATION OF PARTOGRAM _1100h_

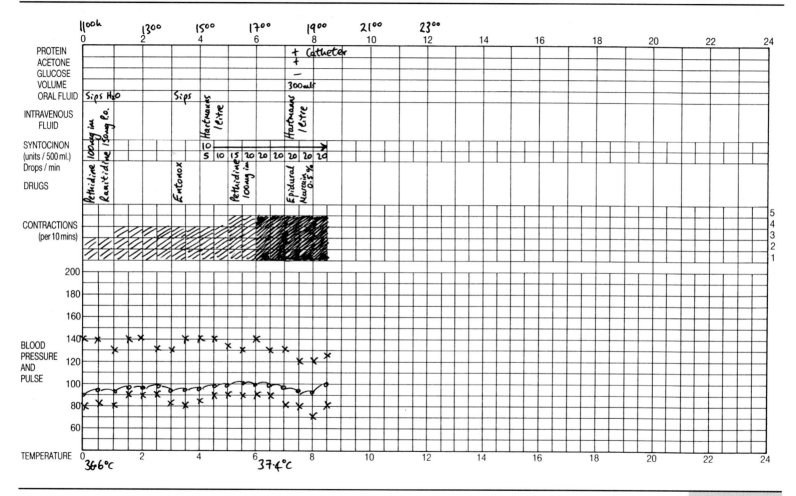

# Outcome

19:30    8 cm, head 2/5 palpable
Caput ++, moulding ++
Right occipito-posterior (ROP)
position

Emergency caesarean section for
secondary arrest in labour
ROP position
3.46 kg male
Apgars 8/1 10/5

The partogram was started too late.
Amniotomy should have been performed
earlier, both to assess the nature of the
liquor and determine the position of the
head. It also allows for more efficient
contractions around the fetal 'pole' (see
page 132).

**22.1**
Baseline 150–170 bpm, good variability,
two shallow Type 2 decelerations (Y).

**22.2**
Baseline 140 bpm; reduced variability;
shallow Type 1 decelerations.

# Clinical points

## STATION AND POSITION OF THE HEAD

It was unfortunate that the position of the head was not determined at any of the vaginal examinations until the final assessment prior to caesarean delivery. This would have provided information as to the reason for the slow labour and would have suggested earlier use of an epidural to provide adequate analgesia—two doses of pethidine were insufficient and a long labour with an occipito-posterior position could have been predicted. Also, in an obstructed labour it becomes increasingly difficult to define the position when caput and moulding develop, obscuring the suture lines and fontanelles.

## ABDOMINAL EXAMINATION

It is vital to examine the maternal abdomen prior to vaginal examination, as the latter may give a false impression of the descent of the fetal head, especially when there is caput. Even had this case reached full dilatation, abdominal delivery would still have been mandatory if the head remained palpable by 2/5 or more.

## CTG PRIOR TO CAESAREAN SECTION

When a patient is taken to theatre it is vital to take the CTG machine and continue to monitor the fetal heart until the operation starts.

## INTRAVENOUS FLUIDS IN LABOUR: 1

Ketonuria may be seen as a physiological occurrence in pregnancy, due to increased fat metabolism. Muscle activity and starvation also result in ketonuria, and so this is commonly seen during labour. As previously discussed (page 23), the partogram enables the recording of fluid balance and urinalysis. Other signs of dehydration in labour include tachycardia, pyrexia, vomiting and a dry tongue. Theoretically labour should not be long enough to allow this to develop, but the mother may have a pre-existing illness, or the ambient temperature may be too high. Even in the absence of dehydration, intravenous fluids are often required, either as a vehicle for drugs, to maintain fluid volume when using an epidural, or when the mother is unable to take an adequate fluid intake orally.

*Cross references:* **Epidurals** *pages 33, 40, 99* **Eating in labour** *page 127* **Amniotomy** *page 132* **Intravenous fluids** *page 187*

# Clinical points

## USING THE CTG ALONE IN INTRAPARTUM MONITORING

In the cases described so far we have relied solely upon the CTG as an indicator of fetal health during labour. A knowledge of antepartum obstetric history combined with the results of other investigations (ultrasound scans, biophysical profile, Doppler waveform studies, etc.) helps to individualize each case. For example, a fetus that has been compromised by chronic placental insufficiency may have adapted to such an extent that its heart rate has compensated and the CTG appears normal. However, such a fetus may not tolerate the additional rigours of labour and the CTG may deteriorate. From the antenatal history it may be possible to determine whether this deterioration is an acute event or a culmination of longer term fetal compromise. However, this may be difficult to establish by looking at the CTG alone, and unfortunately deficiencies in fetal well-being often remain undetected antenatally.

The aim of fetal monitoring is to detect abnormalities at a time when intervention can prevent permanent damage, whether before or during labour. Intrapartum monitoring should be reliable enough to indicate that labour may either be safely allowed to continue, or be terminated. The CTG does not always fulfil this role and often leads to unnecessary intervention, and indeed has been shown to have caused an increase in the caesarean section rate. In most instances sampling fetal blood to assess pH and oxygenation improves the accuracy of intrapartum monitoring, but this does not always provide all the answers (see Cases 23–25).

## INTRAVENOUS FLUIDS IN LABOUR: 2

Hartmann's solution is probably the best intravenous fluid, although normal saline is little different. Dextrose should be avoided as, although it may correct the maternal ketosis, it leads to maternal and fetal hyponatraemia, hyperglycaemia (hence neonatal hyperinsulinaemia and hypoglycaemia) and acid–base imbalance.

# CASE 23

44-year married, Polish secretary

G3 P0 +2 (TOPs)

26.3.91 Admitted via casualty with abdominal pain
Did not know she was pregnant—thought she was menopausal

36-week size uterus, non-tender, contracting
Single fetus, cephalic presentation
Head 2/5 palpable

10:15 Cervix effaced
3 cm dilated, clear liquor

14:00 Head 1/5 palpable
Cervix 6 cm dilated
Left occipito-transverse (LOT) position

16:30 Vaginal examination for fetal blood sampling (FBS)
Still 6 cm, LOT
Clear liquor
Oxytocin started
Pethidine given

19:30 Repeat FBS
8 cm, LOT
Intrauterine pressure catheter (IUPC) inserted

21:00 Fully dilated
Left occipito-anterior (LOA) position
Vertex 1 cm below ischial spines, no moulding
Repeat FBS

# 23.1

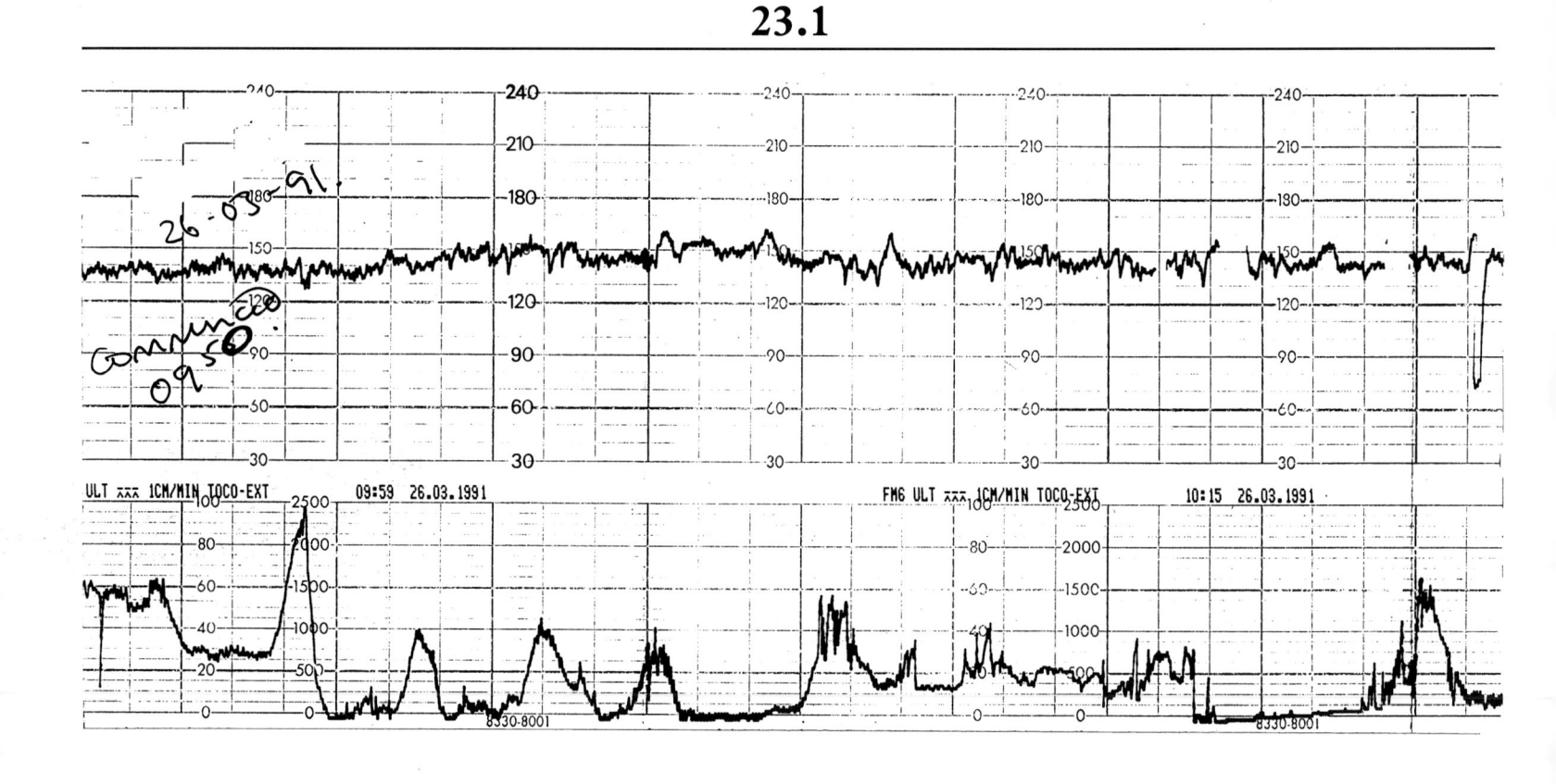

*See page 184 for outcome*

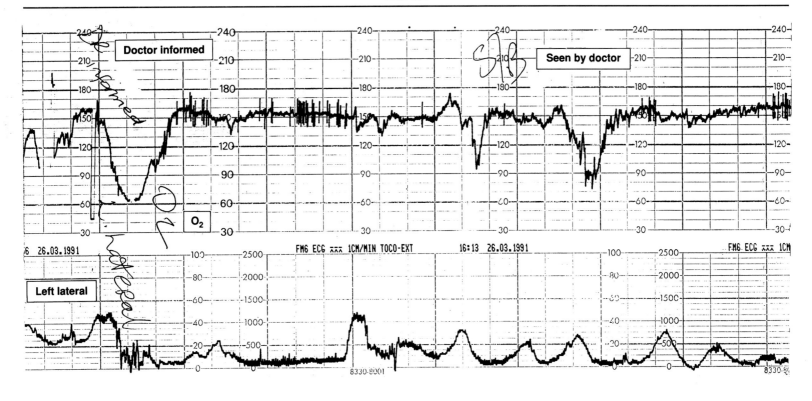

Doctor informed

O₂

Seen by doctor

Left lateral

26.03.1991

FM6 ECG ≈≈≈ 1CM/MIN TOCO-EXT    16:13 26.03.1991

FM6 ECG ≈≈≈ 1CM

8330-8001

*See page 184 for outcome*

CASE 23

# 23.3

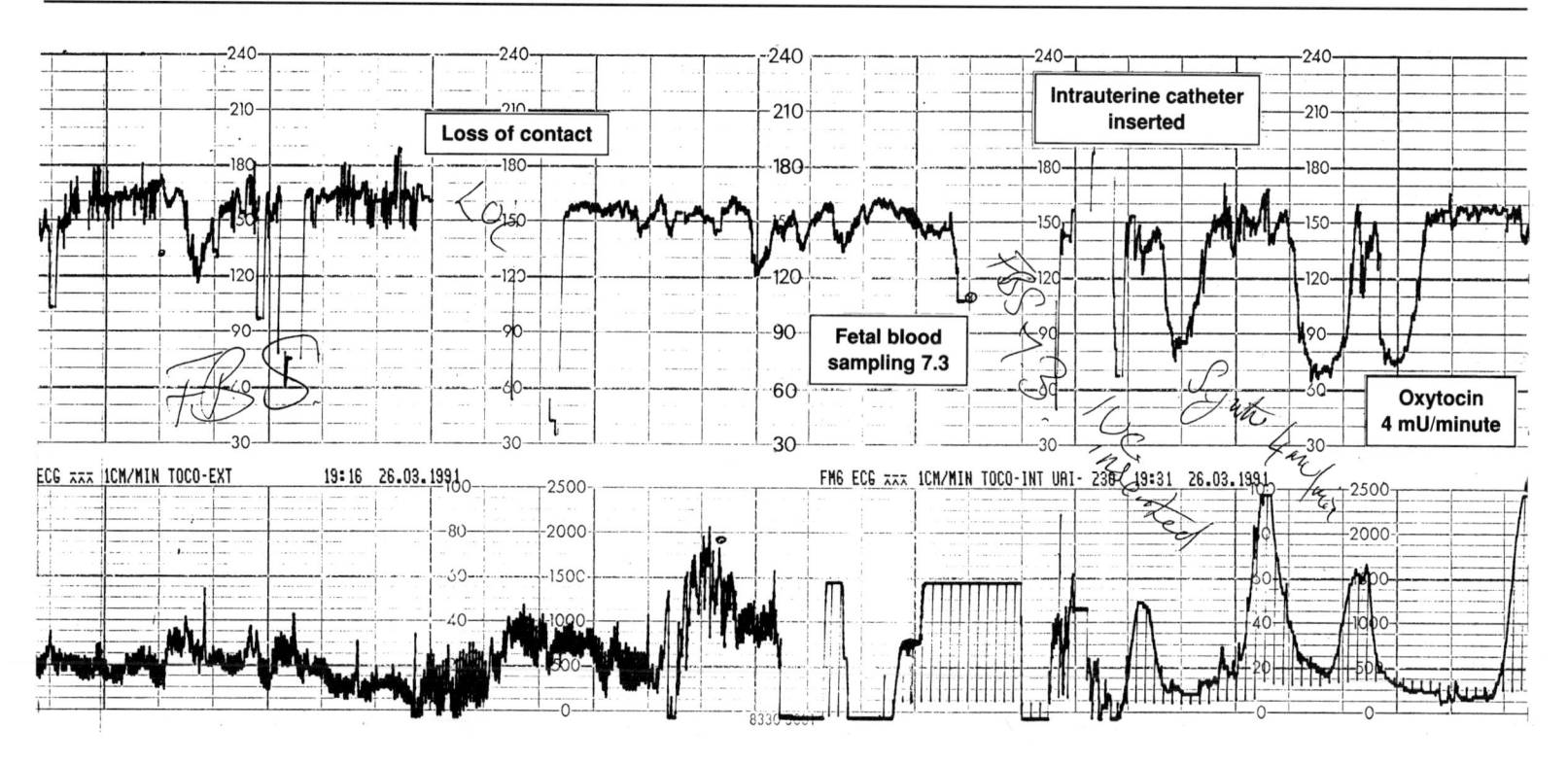

Loss of contact

Intrauterine catheter
inserted

Fetal blood
sampling 7.3

Oxytocin
4 mU/minute

ECG ≈≈ 1CM/MIN TOCO-EXT     19:16  26.03.1991          FM6 ECG ≈≈ 1CM/MIN TOCO-INT UAI- 230 19:31 26.03.1991

*See page 184 for outcome*

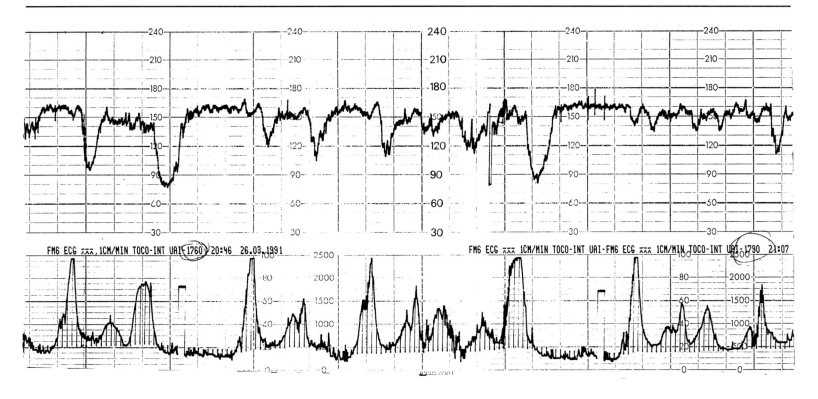

FM6 ECG ⌇⌇⌇ 1CM/MIN TOCO-INT UA1 1760 20:46 26.03.1991    FM6 ECG ⌇⌇⌇ 1CM/MIN TOCO-INT UA1 FM6 ECG ⌇⌇⌇ 1CM/MIN TOCO-INT UA1 1790 21:07

*See page 184 for outcome*

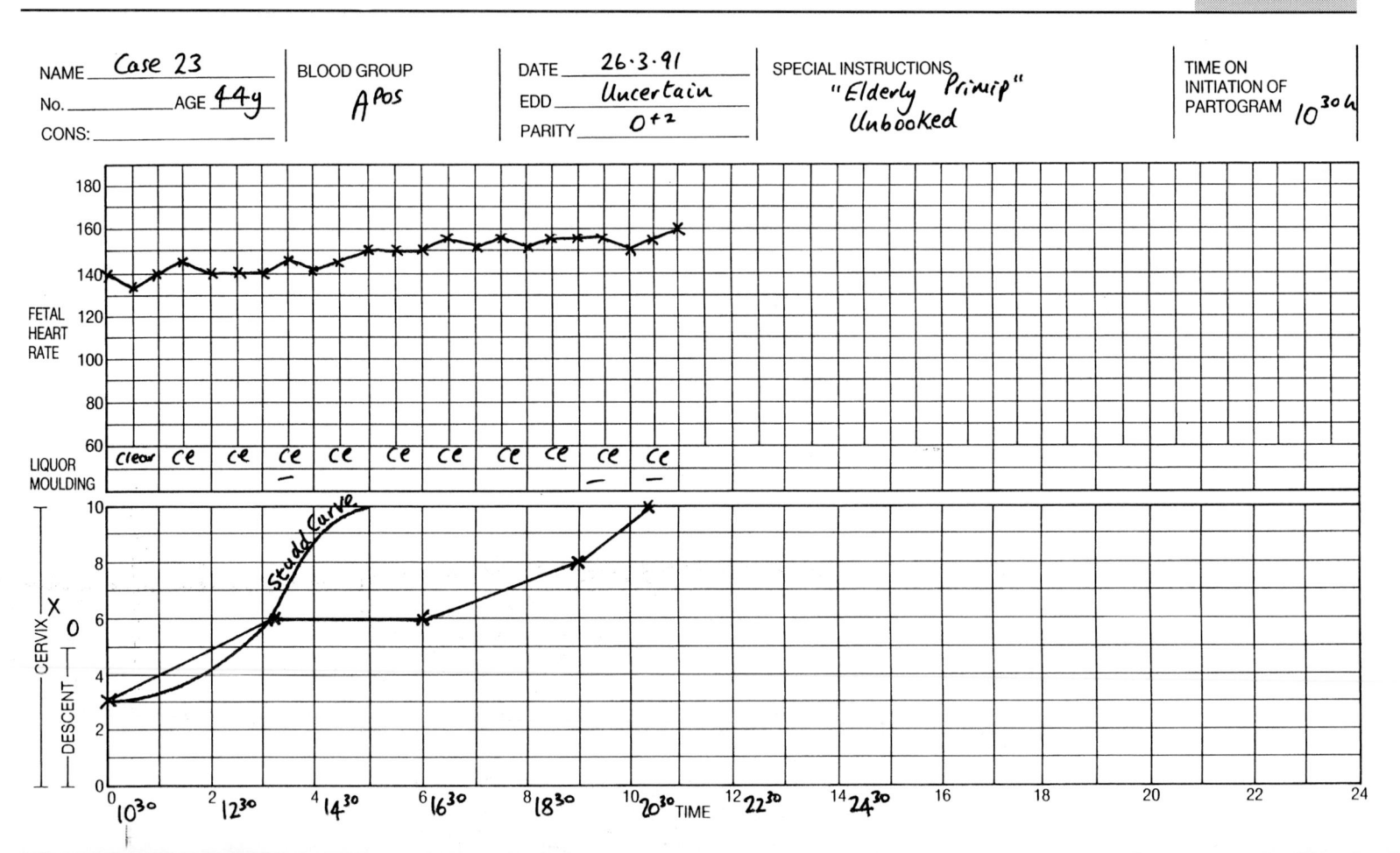

NAME __Case 23__

No. _____ AGE __44y__

CONS: _____

BLOOD GROUP
__A pos__

DATE __26·3·91__

EDD __Uncertain__

PARITY __0+2__

SPECIAL INSTRUCTIONS
"Elderly Primip"
Unbooked

TIME ON
INITIATION OF
PARTOGRAM __10³⁰h__

FETAL
HEART
RATE

180
160
140
120
100
80
60

LIQUOR | Clear | CC | CC | CC | CC | CC | CC | CC | CC | CC | CC
MOULDING | | | | — | | | | | | — | —

CERVIX X
DESCENT O

10
8
6
4
2
0

Studd Curve

TIME

0  10³⁰  2 12³⁰  4 14³⁰  6 16³⁰  8 18³⁰  10 20³⁰  12 22³⁰  14 24³⁰  16  18  20  22  24

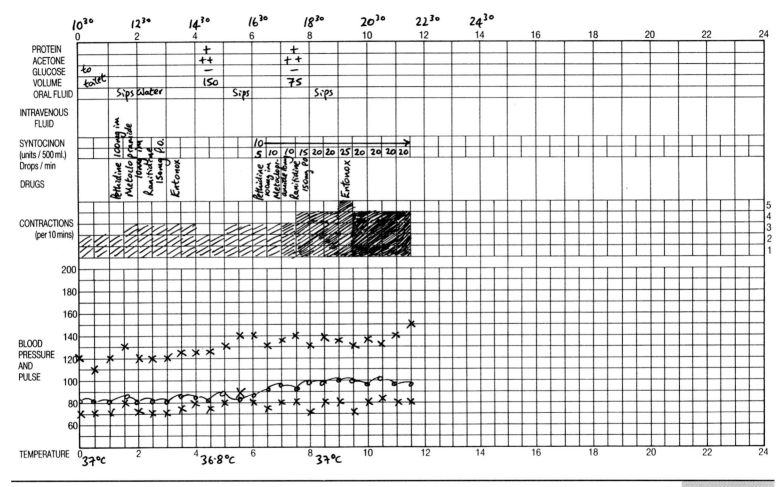

# Outcome

21:45    Normal delivery
          3.45 kg female
          Apgars 8/1 10/5

| Cord gases: | venous | arterial |
|---|---|---|
| pH | 7.32 | 7.30 |
| $pO_2$ (mmHg) | 32 | 21 |
| $pCO_2$ (mmHg) | 40 | 54 |
| Base deficit (mmol/l) | 4.5 | 5.1 |

**23.1**
Baseline 140 bpm. Good variability. A satisfactory trace.

**23.2**
6 hours later, with little progress and an occipito-transverse position, there are signs of discoordinate uterine activity. The baseline heart rate is 150 bpm. The vertical lines are artefactual and tend to mask a reduction in variability. There is one deep and two shallower Type 2 decelerations.

Fetal blood sampling (FBS): pH 7.32, $pO_2$ 24 mmHg, $pCO_2$ 48 mmHg, base deficit 3.8 mmol/l. This is normal, and it is safe to allow labour to continue.

**23.3**
The CTG continues much the same, with a slight rise in baseline rate and occasional Type 2 decelerations. A repeat FBS gives a pH of 7.30, $pO_2$ 24 mmHg, $pCO_2$ 50 mmHg and base deficit of 5.6 mmol/l. An IUPC was inserted at this stage.

**23.4**
The baseline rate continues at 160 bpm. There are a few accelerations, but Type 2 decelerations of varying depth predominate. The uterine activity integral (UAI) is 1760–1790 kPa per 15 minutes. The FBS is: pH 7.28, $pO_2$ 20 mmHg, $pCO_2$ 52 mmHg and base deficit 7.6 mmol/l. These are still within normal limits, but indicate a trend towards hypoxaemia. Since the previous vaginal examination there had been satisfactory progress and the baby delivered shortly afterwards.

This case demonstrates that the FBS may be normal in spite of a persistently worrying CTG trace—indeed, the reassurance provided by the FBS allowed safe augmentation with oxytocin and a normal delivery. This was a high-risk pregnancy in an 'elderly' (i.e. over 35-year) women in her first term pregnancy, who in addition was unbooked and had received no antenatal care.

# Clinical points

Fetal blood sampling is most easily performed with the mother in the left lateral position and her partner sitting on the bed beside her, supporting her upper (right) leg. The procedure can be painful and so analgesia should be provided, for example entonox (50% nitrous oxide + 50% oxygen).

Under aseptic conditions a conical amnioscope is inserted into the vagina and pressed against the fetal head. An area of skin is exposed by pushing the hair to one side and clearing away liquor with a cotton wool bud. Ethyl chloride is sprayed onto a small area. After 1–2 minutes this causes a reactive hyperaemia in the scalp capillaries. Scalp skin has a slow metabolic rate and thus capillary blood provides a good approximation to arterial blood.

Petroleum jelly is applied to the scalp area to encourage droplet formation and a small incision is made. A fine glass capillary is then used to draw up the blood, after which pressure is applied to stop bleeding whilst an assistant takes the sample to be analysed. The results should be ready within 5 minutes.

Normal values for intrapartum capillary samples are:

**pH** : greater than 7.30
**pO$_2$** : greater than 20 mmHg (2.6 kPa)
**pCO$_2$**: less than 50 mmHg (8 kPa)
**base deficit**: less than 8 mmol/l (sometimes termed 'base excess' and recorded as a negative figure)

The pH may be reduced with a respiratory acidosis, a metabolic acidosis or with both together. An abnormal base deficit reflects the metabolic acidosis of anaerobic metabolism, which is secondary to critical hypoxaemia (see lactic acidosis, page 191). A normal base deficit with a low pH suggests respiratory acidosis, which is a state of relatively acute distress in the presence of adequate oxygenation for aerobic metabolism. When there is metabolic acidosis there is also often an element of respiratory acidosis, as evidenced by an elevated pCO$_2$. The overall fetal condition may be assessed by remembering that an abnormal base deficit indicates critical hypoxaemia.

If the pH is less than 7.20 the baby should be delivered; if it is between 7.20–7.25 and it is felt that it is otherwise safe to allow labour to continue, the FBS must be repeated after 30 minutes. A pH of 7.25–7.30 is suspicious and warrants repeat sampling to ensure that the trend is not towards hypoxaemia and acidosis.

*Cross references:* **Cord gases** *page 192* **Fetal blood sampling: 2** *page 186* **Lactic acidosis** *page 192*

# Clinical points

## INTRAUTERINE PRESSURE CATHETER

The use of an IUPC has been discussed in Case 17 (page 132). This may take the form of a fluid-filled tube which is attached to an external transducer that has to be placed at the same level as the intrauterine tip of the catheter. Alternatively, one may use an electronic catheter with the transducer at its tip, as in this case. The latter is more sensitive and is free from the problem of becoming blocked.

The UAI is automatically calculated and is a measure of the area under the contraction curve, expressed in kilopascals per 15 minutes. The average uterine activity is 700–1500 kPa/15 minutes. When oxytocin is being used one should aim for 1000–1500 kPa/15 minutes. A pressure rising above 2000 kPa/15 minutes suggests hyperstimulation with oxytocin or some degree of obstructed labour; women who are grand multiparas or who have a uterine scar are then at risk of uterine rupture unless action is taken to stop oxytocin and/or deliver the baby.

## FETAL BLOOD SAMPLING: 2

An acceleration in the fetal heart rate at the time of FBS is a sign of well-being. It has been suggested by some that if an acceleration is elicited by simply applying pressure to the fetal head, it is then no longer necessary to proceed to blood sampling. Although this approach has some logic, it is not usually employed.

*Cross references:*  **Contraction monitoring** *page 132*  **Fetal blood sampling: 1** *page 185*

# CASE 24

21-year married receptionist

Primigravida

LMP 16.7.90—EDD 23.4.91

Uneventful pregnancy

19.4.91 39+ weeks

21:30   Admitted contracting
       Cephalic presentation
       Head 3/5 palpable
       Cervix effaced, 2 cm dilated
       Membranes intact

20.4.91

00:30   Stronger contractions
       Head 3/5 palpable

01:30   Cervix 4 cm dilated
       Amniotomy, Grade III meconium
       Head 2 cm above ischial spines
       Unable to perform fetal blood
       sampling (FBS)
       Fetal scalp electrode applied
       Epidural sited

03:30   Head 0/5 palpable
       Cervix fully dilated
       Direct occipito-anterior position
       Fetal blood sample obtained

# 24.1

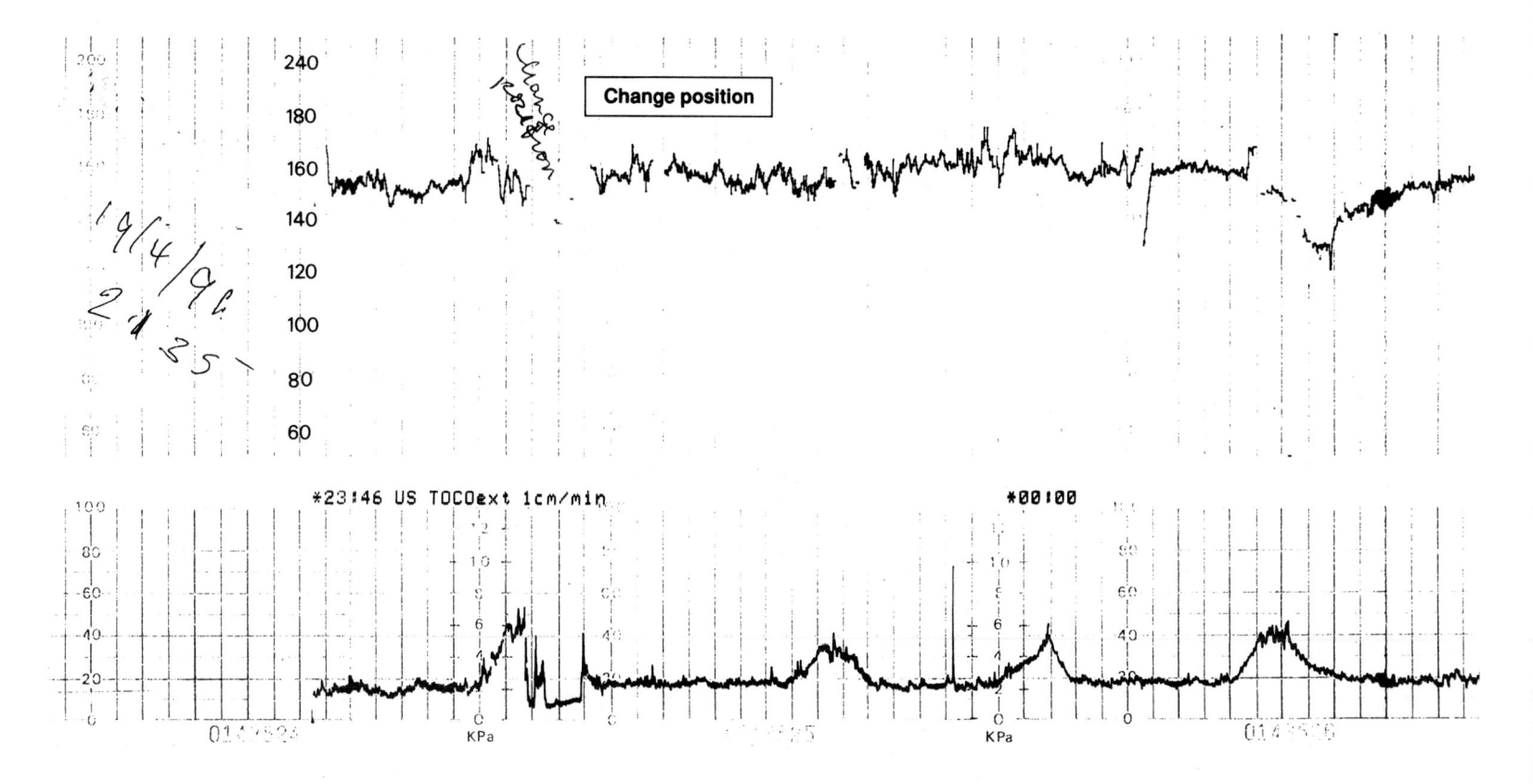

*See page 191 for outcome*

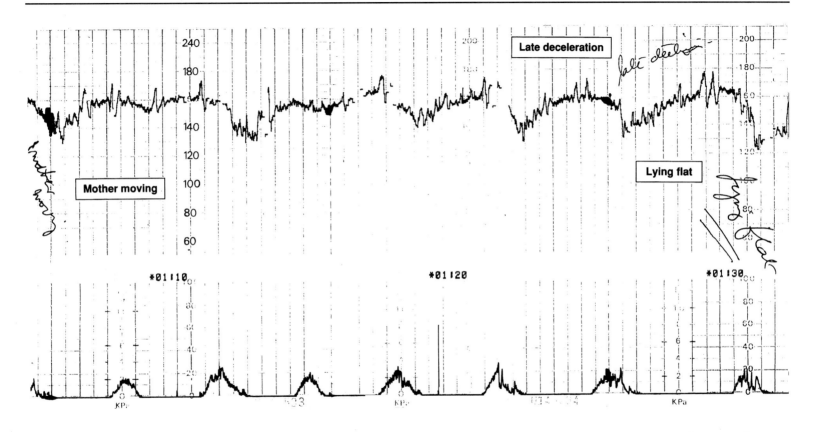

Late deceleration

Mother moving

Lying flat

*01•10

*01•20

*01•30

*See page 191 for outcome*

## 24.3

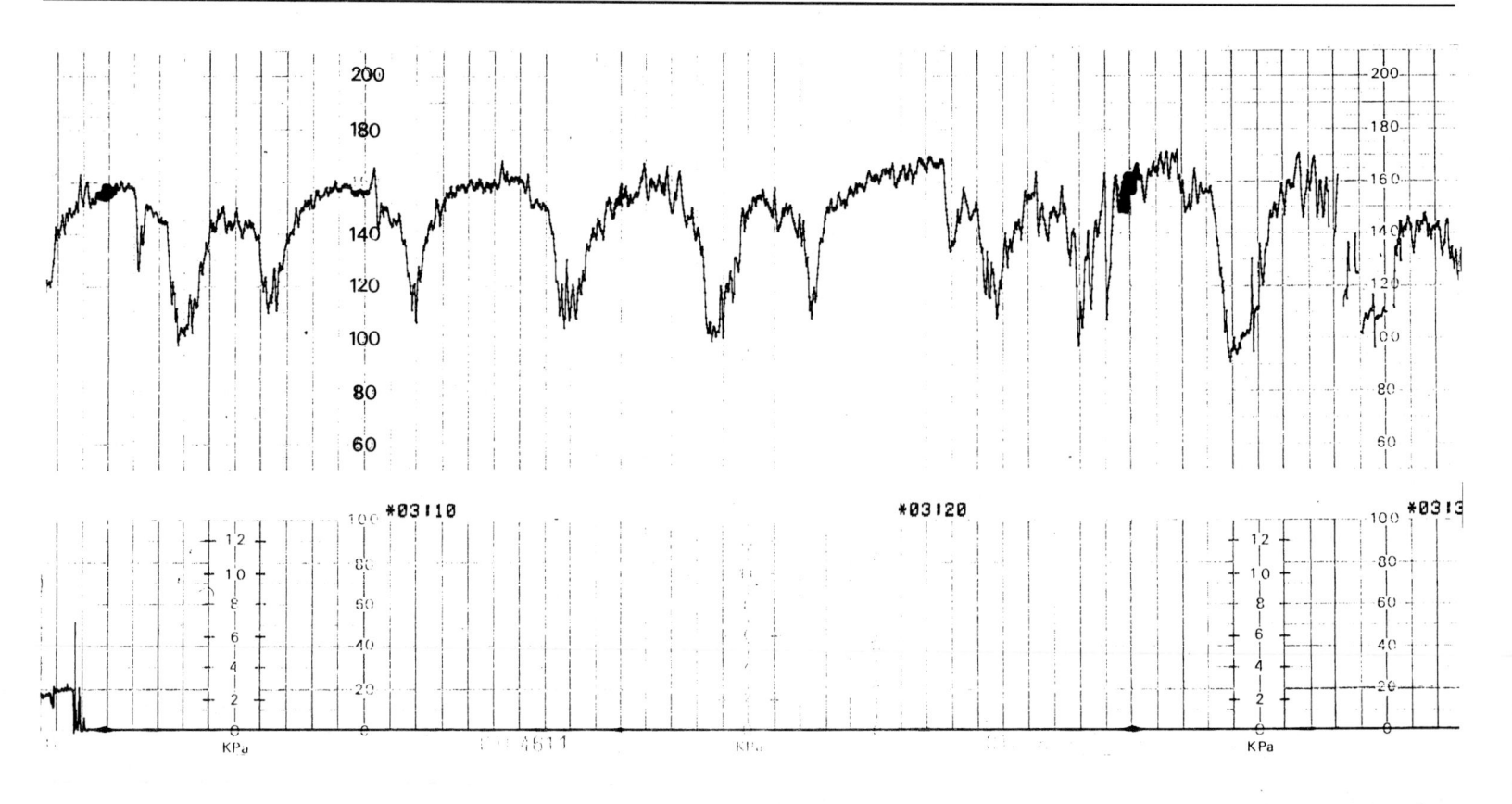

# Outcome

Fetal blood sample:

| | |
|---|---|
| pH | 7.16 |
| pO$_2$ | 15 mmHg |
| pCO$_2$ | 57 mmHg |
| Base deficit | 6 mmol/l |

03:45    Neville–Barnes forceps delivery
3.60 kg male
Apgars 8/1 9/5 10/10—oxygen was
given for the baby to breath, but
no active resuscitation was
required; the baby remained well.

No partogram was kept.

**24.1**
With a baseline rate of 150 bpm there is good variability and Type 2 deceleration.

**24.2**
The baseline rate is 160 bpm. There are persistent Type 2 decelerations and good variability. For technical reasons an FBS could not be taken.

**24.3**
The Type 2 decelerations are deeper. There are no marks to indicate the timing of the contractions. The FBS at this time revealed acute fetal acidosis, and as labour had progressed rapidly an easy outlet forceps delivery was performed and a healthy baby that had no neonatal problems delivered.

Fetal blood sampling was indicated in this case because of both the Grade 3 meconium and the persistent Type 2 decelerations. The procedure may be technically difficult in early labour if the head is high or the cervix less than 4 cm dilated. If blood cannot be obtained one should act on the CTG alone and try again when the cervix has dilated further.

# Clinical points

## CORD GASES

Once the baby has delivered it is useful to examine umbilical arterial and venous gases. The cord should be clamped and the blood analysed within 20 minutes. Cord gases are useful to both obstetrician and paediatrician as they indicate the level of oxygenation and acidosis at the moment of delivery, and the base deficit provides information about the previous 20–30 minutes. Normal values are:

Cord gases should be measured if FBS has been performed during labour, if there has been an operative delivery (instrumental or caesarean) for fetal distress or if there are any worries about fetal condition. The results must be carefully recorded in the notes. Remember that there should be two umbilical arteries and one vein—it is easy to be confused after the excitement of a delivery!

|                   | Venous    | Arterial  |
|-------------------|-----------|-----------|
| pH                | 7.26–7.40 | 7.24–7.35 |
| $pO_2$ (mmHg)     | 24–32     | 14–22     |
| $pCO_2$ (mmHg)    | 33–51     | 40–65     |
| Base deficit (mmol/l) | 2–8   | 2–8       |

## LACTIC ACIDOSIS

pH is determined by a combination of carbon dioxide and lactic acid concentrations. Lactic acid is produced as a consequence of anaerobic metabolism and accumulates during hypoxia, when it may result in cerebral oedema. Lactate levels change fairly slowly and when greater than 4 mmol/l chronic hypoxia has occurred. This assay is not universally available to those performing fetal blood sampling. A fall in pH may also reflect maternal lactic acidosis, which is a not uncommon consequence of labour. Thus the ideal situation is a dual measurement of fetal and maternal blood gases, pH and lactate levels.

---

*Cross references:* **Meconium** *pages 33, 118* **Intravenous fluids in labour** *pages 175, 176* **Fetal blood sampling** *pages 185, 186*

# CASE 25

37-year married housewife

G6 P5

1984 NVD 3.42 kg boy
1985 NVD 3.85 kg boy
1987 NVD 3.98 kg boy
1988 NVD 4.20 kg boy
1989 NVD 3.94 kg boy,
gestational diabetes

EDD 25.4.91 by scan

Uncertain dates
Booked at 16 weeks

Gestational diabetic. Controlled
initially with diet, and then
with insulin from 24 weeks.
Satisfactory growth rate on
serial scans until 36 weeks,
fall in growth at 38 weeks.
Decision taken to induce labour
at 39 weeks.

17.4.91 Prostaglandin gel administered at 06:00
Intravenous insulin and dextrose
infusion commenced

10:00 Irregular contractions
Cephalic presentation, head 3/5 palpable
Cervix 4 cm dilated
Amniotomy, clear liquor

14:00 Contractions still weak and irregular
Cervical dilation unchanged
Intrauterine pressure catheter inserted
Oxytocin infusion started

19:00 Head 2/5 palpable
Cervix 5 cm dilated
Left occipito-posterior position
Fetal blood sampling (FBS) performed

# 25.1

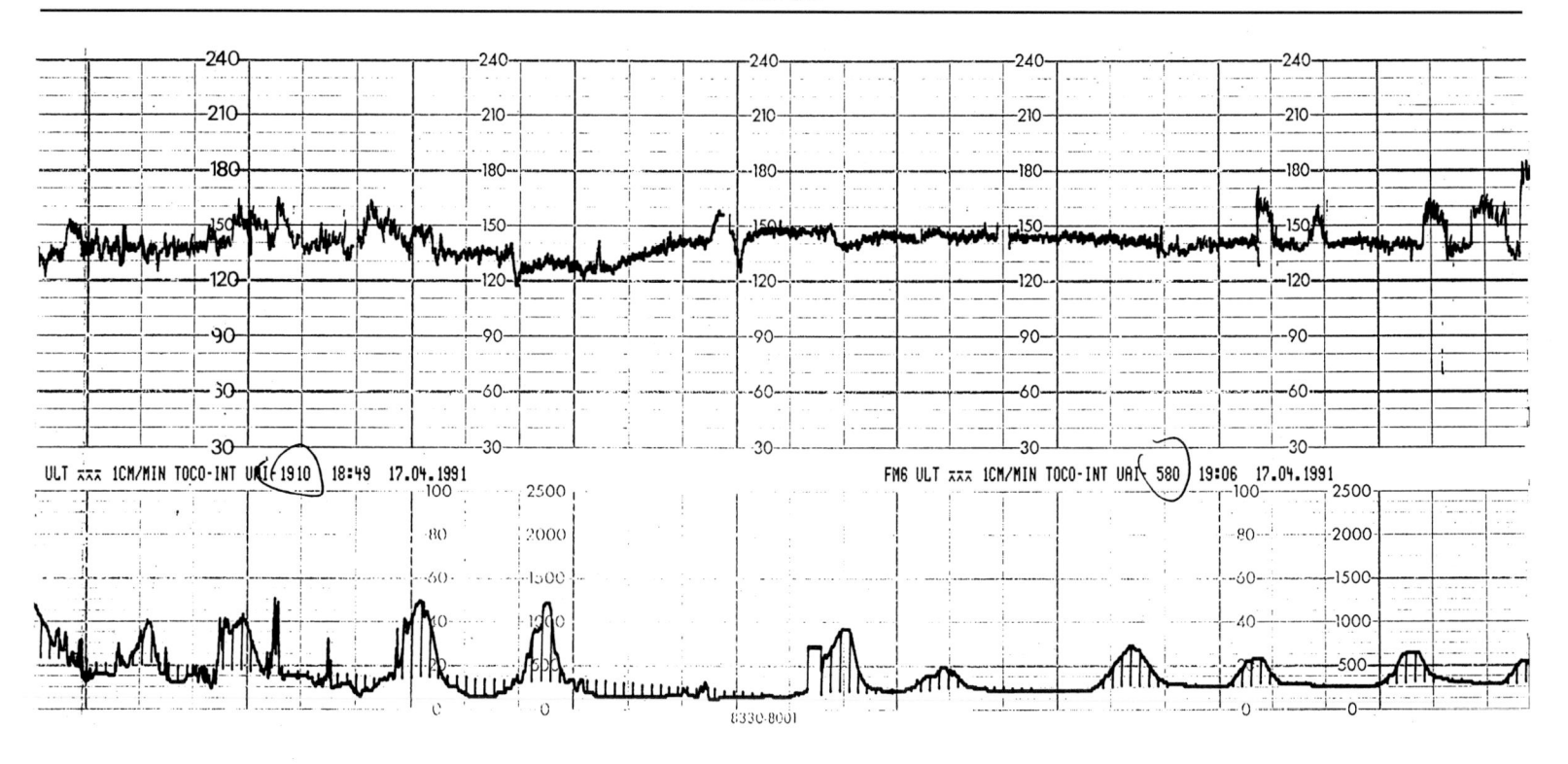

ULT ☵☵ 1CM/MIN TOCO-INT UNIT 1910 18:49 17.04.1991   FM6 ULT ☵☵ 1CM/MIN TOCO-INT UNIT 580 19:06 17.04.1991

*See page 195 for outcome*

# Outcome

Fetal blood sample:

| | |
|---|---|
| pH | 7.16 |
| $pO_2$ | 15 mmHg |
| $pCO_2$ | 57 mmHg |
| Base deficit | 12 mmol/l |

19:30  Emergency caesarean section
3.28 kg female
Apgars 6/1 8/5 10/10

| Cord gases: | venous | arterial |
|---|---|---|
| pH | 7.32 | 7.16 |
| $pO_2$ (mmHg) | 22 | 13 |
| $pCO_2$ (mmHg) | 48 | 60 |
| Base deficit (mmol/l) | 10.5 | 11.4 |

The baby required careful observation in the neonatal period as she became hypoglycaemic, had two apnoeic attacks and then developed jaundice.

No partogram was kept.

## 25.1

The baseline fetal heart rate was 140 bpm and there was reasonable reactivity throughout labour.

It was decided to perform a baseline FBS because of concern about a prolonged, augmented labour in a grand multiparous diabetic mother, in whom there was a worry about fetal growth retardation. An FBS was not strictly warranted as the CTG had been satisfactory, it was therefore surprising to find acidosis and hypoxia severe enough to necessitate immediate delivery. Inspite of having a mother with gestational diabetes, this baby was small compared with its siblings and so the 38-week ultrasound scan had correctly detected placental insufficiency. The baby was in fact quite severely compromised, but it had managed to compensate enough to maintain a normal heart rate.

This case serves to illustrate that there are many aspects to fetal monitoring and no single parameter should be assessed in isolation.

# Conclusion

The CTG is currently the easiest method of obtaining a printed record of fetal condition during labour. But we have demonstrated that it is unwise to rely upon the heart rate alone in determining when the baby should be delivered, whether intrapartum or antenatally. The purpose of any method of fetal monitoring is to identify compromise that will lead to death or morbidity (short- or long-term), so that the cause of the compromise can be corrected, or the fetus liberated from its hostile environment.

The main causes of handicap are chromosomal abnormalities, congenital malformations, intrauterine infection, intrauterine growth retardation (placental insufficiency) and birth trauma—although perinatal events account for less than 10% of cases. Antenatal causes of handicap often remain undetected and so we have become dependent upon intrapartum monitoring to guide us in the management of labour. However, we cannot expect a single variable to predict which babies are at risk of long-term damage.

The CTG has been widely adopted and is used in almost all labour wards. In the increasingly litigious atmosphere of modern obstetrics much store has been put on this printed record as an indicator of the correct management of labour, yet we have tried to show that the CTG does not provide all of the answers. Furthermore, there may be differing opinions on individual traces, and it has been shown that there are wide variations in both intra- and inter-observer interpretations.

The use of electronic fetal monitoring alone does increase the number of caesarean sections performed in labour. The addition of fetal blood sampling (FBS) reduces the caesarian section rate slightly by converting safely some abdominal deliveries into operative vaginal deliveries. We believe FBS to be an essential adjunct for the optimal interpretation of the CTG in labour, and that every labour ward should have the appropriate facilities.

We have shown that no one abnormal fetal heart rate pattern reliably predicts outcome. For example, occasional Type 2 decelerations are more ominous if superimposed on a trace with reduced variability. In order to be able to evaluate the significance of different CTG patterns, one must be aware of the final objective, which is of course long-term infant health. It is therefore unfortunate that the immediate measures of neonatal wellbeing (Apgar scores and cord gases) also correlate poorly with infant handicap! Hypoxic–ischaemic encephalopathy (HIE) describes a range of neurobehavioural states, ranging from mild hyper-excitability to severe hypotonia, the need for ventilation, seizures and coma. Neonatal condition becomes apparent in the first few days of life and, although difficult to quantitate, the degree of HIE provides a better idea of long-term outcome than the early Apgar score.

It is also important to appreciate the ways in which a fetus can adapt to a hostile environment. Long-term placental insufficiency, and hence chronic hypoxia, may result in a compensatory elevation in heart rate such that a superimposed acute hypoxic event does not cause the expected bradycardia. Furthermore, a degree of acidaemia is a physiological adaptation to hypoxia in labour, and so the combination of hypoxia with a normal pH is a poor sign. Great care must thus be taken in correctly interpreting a scalp blood sample.

Continuous intrapartum fetal heart rate recording was widely introduced in the 1960s and 1970s, at a time when national perinatal death rates were also falling. A causal relationship has never been proven, indeed the downwards trend in the perinatal mortality rate had been well established before the introduction of the new technology. There is a significantly decreased incidence of neonatal seizures when continuous fetal heart rate monitoring is used in labours that are abnormal (i.e. induced, augmented or prolonged) rather than 'physiological'. Neonatal seizures are not always associated with long-term handicap, and this again relates to the degree of HIE.

The alternative to continuous monitoring is intermittent auscultation of the fetal heart performed every 15–20 minutes, both during and in between contractions. This is best achieved with a hand-held ultrasound monitor audible to both midwife and parents. It has been shown that this form of monitoring is as effective as continuous monitoring and, if abnormalities are detected, a switch to the latter (and/or FBS) may then take over.

The main implication of intermittent auscultation is the requirement of the individual attention of one midwife to one woman in labour. Sadly, flexible staffing levels of this order are rarely seen in obstetric units in the United Kingdom, and there is little doubt that continuous heart rate monitoring has been used (or rather abused) to allow one midwife to 'care for' two or more women in labour. This practice undermines the important concepts of continuity of care and support in labour.

The CTG does play an important role in fetal monitoring, but it should be remembered that it is a measure of only one parameter of fetal physiology and should be considered in the context of a full appraisal of other events and investigations during both pregnancy and labour. Continuous intrapartum fetal monitoring increases caesarean section rates (and hence maternal morbidity and mortality) without significantly decreasing perinatal mortality or morbidity in low risk labours. If staffing levels are sufficient to permit one-to-one care, intermittent auscultation is preferable in normal, low-risk labours (provided that a baseline CTG in early labour is normal). Continuous monitoring, complemented by fetal blood sampling, should be reserved for higher risk labours (see page 90, case 11).

Whilst research continues in the development of reliable methods of fetal assessment that aim to predict long-term outcome, the recording of the fetal heart rate continues to be a simple means of intrapartum monitoring. Yet only a judicious use of the CTG enables us to best care for each mother and her baby.

# Further reading

Chalmers I, Enkin M, Keirse M J N C (eds) 1989 Effective Care in Pregnancy and Childbirth. Oxford University Press, Oxford

Grant A, O'Brien N, Joy M T, Hennesy E, MacDonald D 1989 Cerebral palsy among children born during the Dublin randomised trial of intrapartum monitoring. Lancet ii: 1233–1235

Niswander K R 1991 External Fetal Monitoring and brain damage in term and post-term infants. Contemporary Obstetrics and Gynecology 36: 39–50

Smith J H 1992 Is continuous intrapartum fetal monitoring necessary? In: Chard T, Richards M (eds) Benefits and hazards of the new obstetrics. MacKeith Press, London. In press

Spencer J A D (ed) 1989 Fetal monitoring, physiology and techniques of antenatal and intrapartum assessment. Castle House Publications Ltd, Tunbridge Wells

Wheble A M, Gillmer M D G, Spencer J A D, Sykes G S 1989 Changes in fetal monitoring practices in the UK: 1977–84. British Journal of Obstetrics and Gynaecology 96: 1140–1147

# Index

Bold page numbers indicate topics that appear as clinical discussion points.

Abdominal examination, 17, **175**

Acceleration, 3, 6, 81
   examples in cases, 16, 22, 32, 39, 58, 70, 80, 98, 126, 150, 156, 166

Acidosis (see hypoxia)
   metabolic, 185
   respiratory, 185

Action line, 17

Amniotomy (see rupture of membranes)
   with polyhydramnios, **114**

Anaemia, 2, 3

Analgesics, 3

Antacids in labour, **127**

Antenatal CTG, **49**, **81**

Antenatal monitoring, **45**, 49, 59, 71, 81, 86

Antihypertensive drugs, 1, 3, 7, 70

Apgar scores, **167**, 168, 196

Artefact, 3, 8, 98

Asphyxia (see fetal asphyxia)

Augmentation (see oxytocin)

Base deficit, 185, 192

Baseline
   falling, 7, 16, 22
   rate, 17, 81, 32
   variability, 1, 2, 3, 6, 49, 81

Beat-to-beat variability (see variability)

Biochemical tests, **59**, 151

Biophysical profile, **86**, 141

Blood pressure, 7

Bradycardia, 1, 32, 58, 108, 150, 156

Breech presentation, 117, **118**, 167

Caesarean section (see delivery)

Cardiac arrhythmias, 2

Cardiotocograph (CTG), 1, 86, 90, 196
   alone in intrapartum monitoring, **176**
   antenatal, **49**, **81**
   continuous, **90**, 109, **151**, 197
   intermittent, 90, 197
   prior to caesarean section, **175**
   quality, 8, 126
   terminal, 49, 85
   twin, 141

Catheterisation, **23**

Cephalopelvic disproportion (CPD), 17, 71, 108, 131

Circumcision, **17**